SO-AXJ-267

Fit in
15

Fit in 15

15-minute
morning workouts
that balance
cardio, strength
and flexibility

Steven Stiefel

Photographs by Robert Holmes

Ulysses Press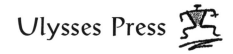

Text Copyright © 2005 Steven Stiefel. Photographs Copyright © 2005 Robert Holmes (all photos on pages not enumerated below). Photographs Copyright © 2005 photos.com (all photos on pages enumerated below). All rights reserved. No part of this publication may be reproduced, stored in a retrieval system, or transmitted in any form or by any means without the prior written permission of the publisher, nor be otherwise circulated in any form of binding or cover other than that in which it is published and without a similar condition being imposed on the subsequent purchaser, except for use by a reviewer in connection with a review.

Published in the United States by
Ulysses Press
P.O. Box 3440
Berkeley, CA 94703
www.ulyssespress.com

ISBN 1-56975-471-3
Library of Congress Control Number 2005922404

Printed in Canada by Transcontinental Printing

10 9 8 7 6 5 4 3 2 1

Editorial/Production	Lily Chou, Claire Chun, Tamara Kowalski, Steven Zah Schwartz, Matt Orendorff
Interior Design	Robles-Aragón
Cover Design	Eleanor Reagh
Photography	Robert Holmes
	Photos.com: pages 8, 10, 11, 12, 13, 14, 16, 17, 18, 20, 26, 27, 28, 29, 32, 35, 36, 37, 43, 49, 50, 51, 52, 53, 56, 59, 60, 61, 62, 65, 130, 138, 140, 141
Front cover photograph	© Getty Images. Stockbyte/Stockbyte Gold Collection
Exercise Models	Rocky Fain, Sonja Soriano, Steven Stiefel, Andrea Alejandro, David Reid

Distributed by Publishers Group West

Please Note
This book has been written and published strictly for informational purposes, and in no way should be used as a substitute for consultation with health care professionals. You should not consider educational material herein to be the practice of medicine or to replace consultation with a physician or other medical practitioner. The author and publisher are providing you with information in this work so that you can have the knowledge and can choose, at your own risk, to act on that knowledge. The author and publisher also urge all readers to be aware of their health status and to consult health care professionals before beginning any fitness program.

Part 1: **Overview**

Part 2: **Programs**

Part 3: **Workouts**

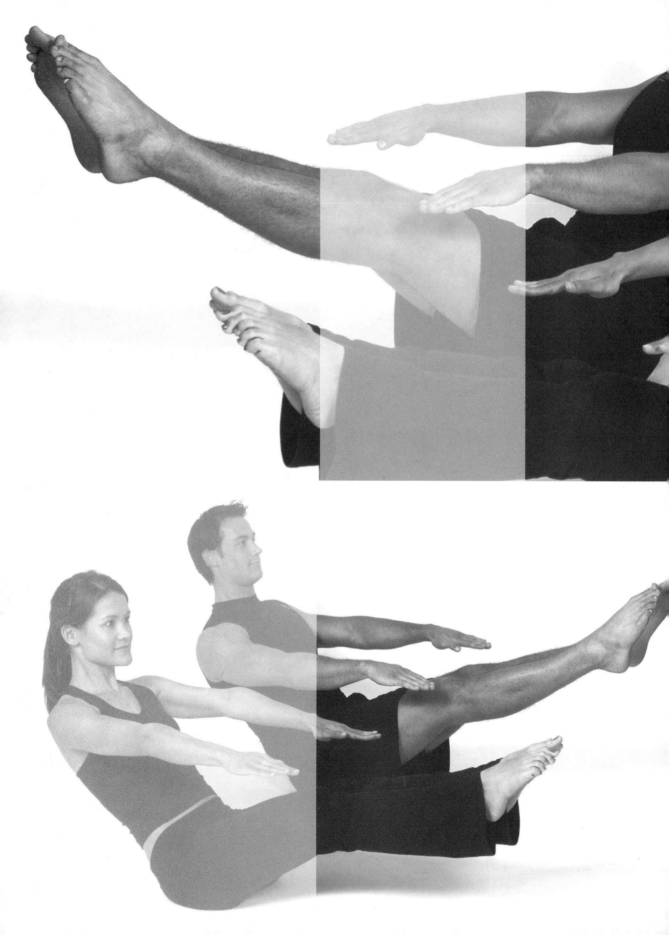

Part

1

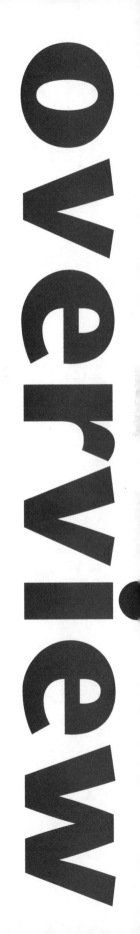

The Fit in 15 Philosophy

Many fitness programs overpromise what you can reasonably expect to achieve from them. They may claim that you can get perfectly defined abs or toned thighs in a couple of weeks by spending only a few minutes here or there. These "miracle plans" are almost always hype to persuade you to buy some gadget that you probably won't use after a week or two, if at all.

Saying that you can get fit in only 15 minutes a day may sound like similar hype, but it's not. The Fit in 15 program allows you to create a reasonable full-fitness program based on your personal goals. If you can devote 15 minutes every day to exercising first thing in the morning, you'll be surprised by not only how fit you will get, but by how much better you will look and feel.

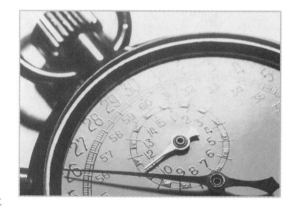

The biggest difference between these trendy fads that don't work and the Fit in 15 program is that Fit in 15 asks you to make a commitment that you will be happy to make. On the Fit in 15 program, you'll be creating your own relationship with your fitness and health. Once you start this relationship, you'll begin to get results, which will motivate you to continue spending a few minutes every morning with your Fit in 15 program.

The Fit in 15 Program

The Fit in 15 program, unlike most programs on the market, target-trains your body for full fitness by involving strength, core, target (to work on trouble spots), mind/body and flexibility training. Each workout is performed on a specific day of the week, giving you a quick yet comprehensive personalized exercise program.

Many people who exercise regularly follow the same regimen day in, day out. While regular activity of any sort—whether it's walking for 15 minutes, weight

FIT IN 15 SCHEDULE

MONDAY:	Cardiovascular Training
TUESDAY:	Strength Training—Upper Body & Core
WEDNESDAY:	Flexibility Training
THURSDAY:	Strength Training—Lower Body & Core
FRIDAY:	Cardiovascular Training
SATURDAY:	Target Training
SUNDAY:	Mind/Body Training

training for 20 minutes, using a treadmill for 30 minutes—is far better than no activity at all, it can get a little dull. Also, performing the same activity every day doesn't make you fully fit because you're only working your body in one particular way each time you train. The Fit in 15 program teaches you how to train your body for all the different elements of fitness, above and beyond just "physical" fitness when you also factor in the mind/body benefits. Plus, Fit in 15 allows you to individualize your program with target-training workouts, specialized workouts to, among many options, tone your thighs or reduce body fat.

"Full fitness" may sound like you'll be training all the time, but that's not the case. The Fit in 15 program is not a hardcore regimen that will turn you into a pro athlete or muscle-bound bodybuilder. Rather, it's designed for the average person with a busy lifestyle who wants to become fit in a short period of time, without becoming compulsive about it. With a relatively small commitment of only 15 minutes a day, you may be surprised at how much you can accomplish in terms of your health, well-being and physical appearance.

On the other hand, we're not limiting you to only 15 minutes of exercise a day. If you want to do more, you can. As you become more fit, feel free to go above and beyond the workouts described in the Fit in 15 program (see "Continue Your Progress" at the end of the book). In addition, don't forget that an evening walk or activities around the house are also important components to living a fit lifestyle. Add those into your life as often as possible.

Getting Started

In this overview, you're getting a good sense of the philosophy and dynamics of the Fit in 15 program. Part Two describes the various types of fitness training, including core, strength, cardiovascular and flexibility. Acquaint yourself with these elements and decide what you want to achieve. Honestly assess where you are today, and how you can best get to where you want to be. Also, pay particular attention to the Target Training section so that you can construct a program that will really help you meet your goals.

Finally, take a careful look at the range of workout options explained in Part Three. Choose a workout option from each day of the week that's right for you—you might decide to do all the standard programs, or perhaps the less-intense "Easy Does It" workouts. You can also mix and match various styles of workouts. For instance, you might opt for the "Easy Does It" lower-body strength workout while choosing a more demanding workout on your Monday and Friday Cardiovascular Training days.

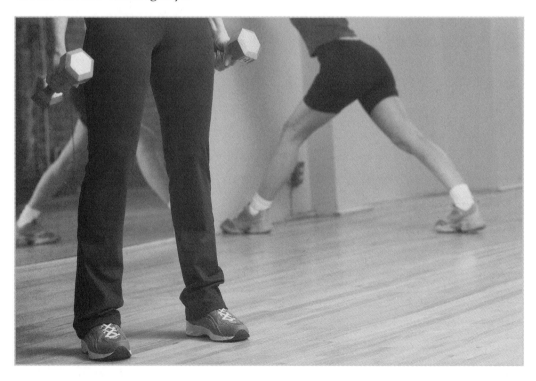

Above all, read through the workout and exercise descriptions and follow the directions carefully. By doing so, you'll help prevent injury as well as get improved results. Once you're comfortable with your basic Fit in 15 program, take a look at "Continue Your Progress" at the end of the book to see how you can continue making further improvements to your program. It includes advice on how to build longer workout programs, how to change up your program and how to use intensity to make the most of your Fit in 15 program.

As you get started, two questions may arise about performing your Fit in 15 program in the morning.

Do I have to do the program first thing in the morning?

You can schedule the program whenever you like, but we've found that people are more likely to stay devoted to their Fit in 15 program if they get up and get to it (some would say "get it out of the way") first thing in the morning. Morning exercise also helps wake you up, rev up your metabolism, and give you energy for the rest of the day. But if you're not a morning person, or not one for morning exercise, other times of day can work just as well. Working out some time during the day is far better than not working out at all.

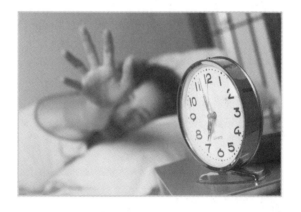

What should I eat before I workout?

Studies show that if you don't eat before you exercise, you're more likely to burn calories from stored fat—a real plus. When you eat first, your body is more likely to turn to the calories you've just consumed for its first source of energy before reaching for stored body fat. Of course, these are tendencies, not absolutes. If you eat a few calories, your body won't avoid burning body fat—it may simply not burn as many of these unwanted stored calories.

Do whichever feels best for your body. Some people feel great when they work out on an empty stomach; others need a little food in their system. If you're going to eat before you perform your Fit in 15 program, then I recommend a small amount of carbs and protein. Here are some good pre-workout choices:

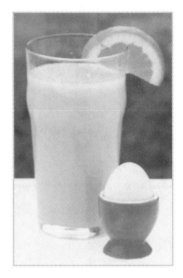

A small glass of juice and a boiled egg

A bagel with light cream cheese

A piece of toast with peanut butter

A piece of fruit and a handful of nuts.

You can also have water or a cup of coffee or tea (with a little sugar or nonfat milk, if desired).

After you work out, eat a healthy, substantive breakfast. Your body will be primed to handle the calories for muscle building, recovery and energy conversion. You've often heard that breakfast is the most important meal of the day. This is part of the reason why it's true.

Equipment

Very little equipment is needed for the Fit in 15 program, although to get the most from the strength-training moves, you really do need at least one pair of dumbbells. The rest of the equipment is truly optional. For the most part, each day's workout plans include a way to work out without equipment, but variations in the workouts may refer to pieces of equipment.

For information on specific equipment and gear that can enhance your workouts, see the individual Equipment sections in Part Two.

Everyday Exercise

Why not just work out for an hour a day twice a week? Isn't that even more exercise than the seven 15-minute sessions in the Fit in 15 program? Here's the answer: Just as you wouldn't eat all your meals for the week on Monday and Tuesday and then skip eating until the next week, it's crucial that you spread your exercise throughout the week to get the most beneficial effects.

Daily exercise has a major impact on your metabolic rate, which can be defined as the amount of calories your body naturally burns in its resting state. When you become more active, your body begins to expend more energy each day for physiological processes such as digestion and sleep. This is one of the biggest advantages of regular exercise.

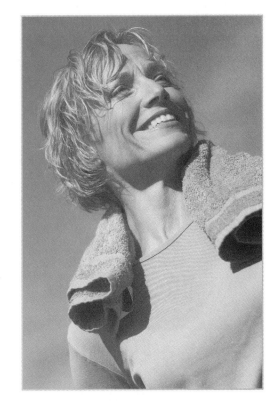

You'll be exercising almost every day for a short period of time. But instead of feeling wiped out, as you may have experienced from long, intense bouts of exercise, the Fit in 15 program will help invigorate you. The immediate response will be an increased metabolic rate, making you feel energized and ready for the rest of your day. And, because the exercise sessions are brief, you'll be far less likely to "crash" later on in the day.

Another important component of exercising every day is that it will become part of your daily routine in the way that a morning shower or breakfast already is. Exercising will become second nature, something that you want to do, something that you do automatically rather than agonizing over whether or not you feel like doing it each morning.

Everyday Nutrition

If one of your Fit in 15 goals is to manage your weight or reduce body fat, then the nutritional component of your program can be as important as the exercise regimen. The following tips will allow you to manage your body weight, as well as increase the amount of body fat you are able to burn each day.

EAT MORE MEALS A DAY.   One of the hardest pieces of nutritional advice to accept is that eating more meals a day will help keep you from adding unwanted body fat. Of course, it seems logical that the fewer times a day that you eat, the less likely

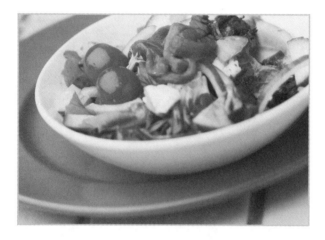

you are to consume enough calories to store as fat. But the body is complex. When you feed it a lot of calories but do so only once or twice a day, you are sending your body the message that food is scarce, and it needs to hoard the little you're giving it. Your body responds by reducing its metabolic rate (the amount of energy it burns each day) and pulling calories into storage as body fat rather than immediately burning them for fuel.

When you eat more meals a day, the opposite happens. You send your body the message that food is plentiful. The process of eating and digesting also increases your metabolic rate (each time you consume a meal, it's like throwing more fuel on a fire). The key is—of course—to keep these multiple meals small enough that you aren't consuming more calories than you were when you were eating fewer meals a day. Ideally, you should eat four to six times a day. Eat small- to moderate-sized meals and have a snack or two throughout the day. Emphasize quality whole foods (see "Eat whole foods" below for details).

AVOID CUTTING CALORIES TOO MUCH. Cutting calories will help you lose weight, but only for the short term. When you cut too many calories for too long, you will slow down your metabolic rate. Then, when you stop your low-calorie diet and start eating a normal amount of food, you will be even more likely to store those calories as body fat because your metabolic rate has been reduced.

A far better strategy is to cut the amount of calories you're consuming each day by only ten percent or so. If you normally consume 2000 calories, then your diet should not go below 1800 calories for the best long-term results. Almost every person with a healthy metabolic rate needs at least 1700 or 1800 calories a day for all their nutritional needs. If you're currently adding body fat at or below this daily calorie-consumption rate, you can improve your metabolic rate through the exercise portion of this program and with these nutrition tips.

CONSUME ADEQUATE PROTEIN. Popular high-protein diets such as the Atkins have their supporters and detractors. Rather than strictly following one of these diets, you can simply consume an adequate amount of protein for your body weight each day while emphasizing whole foods for the bulk of your calories. Use the following guideline for protein consumption:

DAILY PROTEIN CONSUMPTION	
YOUR WEIGHT (pounds)	DAILY PROTEIN NEED (grams)
100	70
125	87
150	105
175	122
200	140
225	157
250	175
275	192
300	210

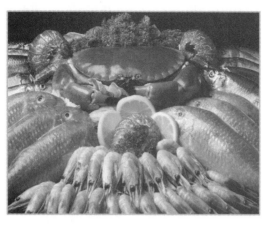

You need protein to keep your body growing and replenishing itself, especially if you are on a fitness program such as Fit in 15. For best results, you should consume more than .7 grams of protein for each pound of body weight. However, every body is unique. We all have physiological quirks. Some people feel great when they rely on meat as a cornerstone of their diet. Others don't process this category of food well at all. For instance, if you're lactose intolerant, avoid excessive amounts of dairy. Pay attention and emphasize the types of foods and the eating strategies that work best for you.

EAT WHOLE FOODS. Emphasizing whole foods in your nutrition program has been mentioned in the previous tips because it's very important. Whole foods are those that are not refined or processed. They are foods that are closest to the way they are found in nature. Excellent whole-food choices come from the following categories:

- Meat and fish
- Dairy (milk and eggs)
- Fruits
- Vegetables
- Nuts and seeds

When the bulk of your diet comes from foods in these categories, you will be providing yourself with a much better nutrient profile than when you eat pre-packaged and refined foods.

DRINK FLUIDS. Consuming plenty of fluids is vital for both health and nutrition. The average adult should drink eight eight-ounce glasses of water a day. Most people fall far short of this, causing dehydration, a condition that creates unnecessary stress on your body. Other liquids such as coffee, tea, juice and even milk have a lot of water in them, and they help stave off dehydration, but no liquid is as healthy for your body as pure water.

REDUCE CONSUMPTION OF OVER-PROCESSED FOODS.   At the same time that you eat healthier whole foods, strive to reduce processed and refined foods. Two of the biggest culprits are bleached flour and refined sugars—two of the most crucial ingredients to many of the best desserts. Notice that the recommendation is to reduce these foods, not eliminate them. You should occasionally include desserts as treats—even on a day-to-day basis, if desired, but in small quantities.

Trans-fats, found in such things as margarine and vegetable shortening, should also be avoided. These man-made fats are not healthy in any way and are far worse than the natural fats found in meat and dairy products.

DON'T OBSESS OVER CARBS AND FAT GRAMS.   Almost all of the diet fads of the past few years suggest cutting carbs, fats or both. The answer: Don't obsess over carbs or fat intake. Follow the above recommendations, and the amounts of fat and carbs in your diet will take care of themselves. Emphasize whole foods, eat plenty of protein, keep your calories moderate, and you can be assured that you will be taking in the right amount of carbs and fats.

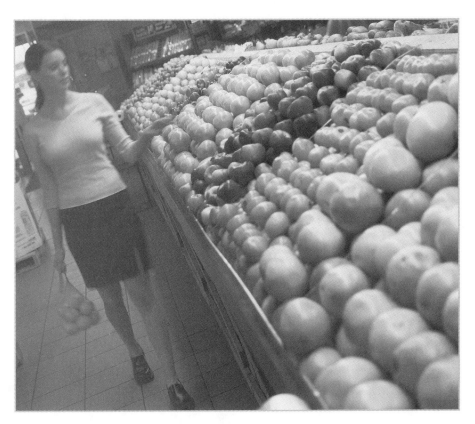

Easy Does It

What if you feel that you are not in good enough shape to start with a full 15 minutes of exercise every day? Or what if you've recently been injured but are trying to get back into shape? Fit in 15 provides an easy-does-it alternative for your Monday-through-Friday workouts.

Before you begin any workout program, it's imperative that you get your doctor's approval. This is particularly true if you are recovering from an injury, are in a high-risk category or suffer from any sort of ongoing condition (such as arthritis, diabetes, heart disease, etc.). Once you have received clearance from your doctor, keep the following points in mind as you begin your Fit in 15 program:

FOLLOW ALL ADVICE AND MODIFICATIONS GIVEN TO YOU BY YOUR DOCTOR. For instance, your doctor may tell you that a particular type of exercise (such as running) is not a good option for you. Heed this advice and choose a more appro-

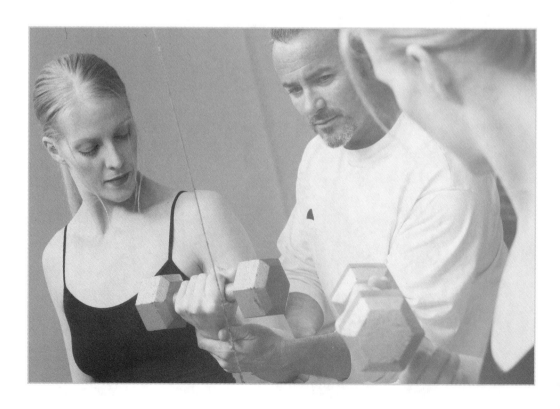

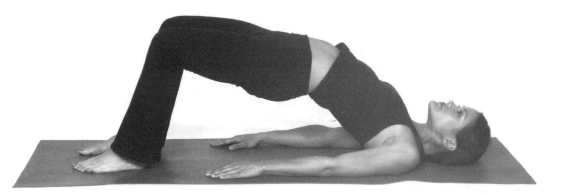

priate workout from the options for that day of the week (such as swimming or walking). If you are told not to do a certain type of exercise at all (such as lower-body strength training), then substitute a workout from another day of the week (such as adding another day of walking to your regimen).

START SLOWLY. You're far better off starting with a program that's a little on the easy side than one that's too hard for you. Often, people get very enthusiastic when they first begin a new program (whether it's a nutritional or exercise one), and they set themselves up for failure by making the program too hard to maintain.

At first, you might feel a little stiff or sore from some of the exercises or work-outs in this book. But if you are so sore that it's almost impossible to do your next day's workout, then you should back off. Lessen the intensity by reducing the amount of weight you use, the number of reps and sets you perform, the length of time you work out, or the amount of energy you bring to your exercise (or some combination of these variables).

ALWAYS GUARD AGAINST INJURY. If your body tells you to slow down or stop, listen. For instance, if your back starts to twitch when you're performing lunges, stop. Don't continue just because the workout chart tells you to. You'll be far better off in the long run responding to the feedback that your body is giving you than you will in pushing past the point of common sense.

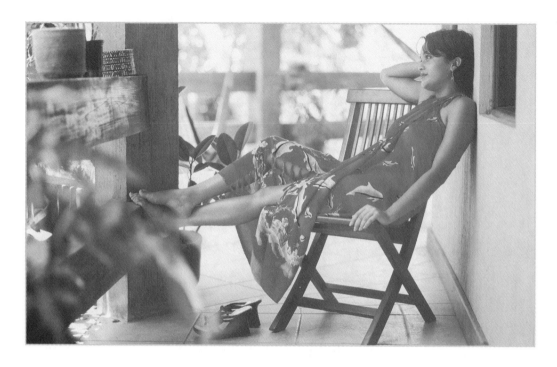

TAKE REST DAYS IF YOU FEEL LIKE YOU'VE TRAINED TOO MUCH RECENTLY. While the Fit in 15 program gives you a workout for every day of the week, you don't necessarily need to work out every day. Remember, your body grows and improves when it is recovering from exercise, not while it is exercising. Exercise itself is a stress on the body, with benefits resulting from how your body learns to adapt to this stress. It learns to adapt in the rest periods following workouts. If your body is overtrained or exhausted (or if you're coming down with a cold or other malady), you are more likely to harm your body than increase your progress by working out when you shouldn't. Again, listen to the feedback from your body. This should always be your guide in deciding when to take a day off.

LEARN HOW TO MONITOR YOUR HEART RATE. Ask your doctor if you should get a heart rate monitor and use it to check your heart rate. Knowing your resting and target heart rates can help you determine if you are engaging in exercise that is appropriate for you.

Easy-Does-It Workouts

With all of the above in mind, you can follow an "Easy Does It" program by exclusively using the Easy-Does-It Workouts, especially when you first begin the Fit in 15 program. Or you can perform Easy-Does-It Workouts only for certain days of the week. For instance, if flexibility is your weakest area of fitness, you may find that easing up on flexibility training is a good idea. Or you can also choose Easy-Does-It Workouts on a day here or there when you don't have as much energy or drive, but would still like to keep with your Fit in 15 routine. Include Easy-Does-It Workouts in your Fit in 15 program as often or as infrequently as desired.

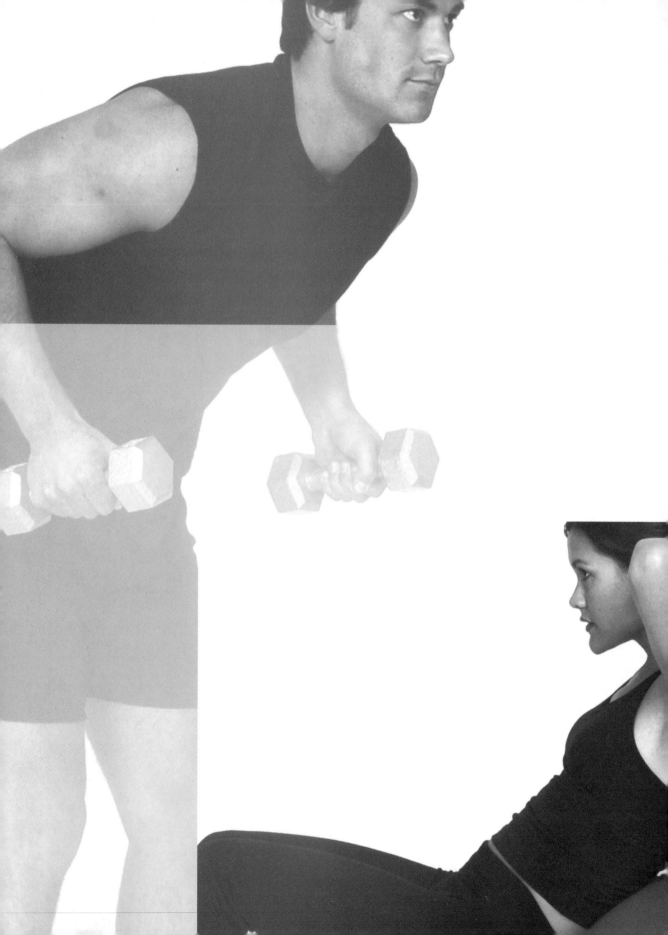

Part 2

programs

Determining Your Levels

To determine whether to choose the Starter or Experienced level, give your current fitness level an honest assessment. If you've worked out regularly in the past but haven't done much in the past few months, you may need to return to the Starter level. Or, if you have an active lifestyle but haven't done focused exercise, you may find that you're in better shape than you expected and you may be able to train at the Experienced level.

Finally, assess your level for each type of fitness, including cardiovascular, strength (both upper- and lower-body) and flexibility. Often, a person will be more advanced in one area, and in need of a slower start in another.

STARTER   People with little or no exercise experience are clearly Starters. But, even if you have exercised in the past, it's a safer bet to start fresh with the Starter level than it is to jump to the Experienced level just because you have past familiarity with a particular type of exercise. You can always move up in a few weeks or a month of two. Starting slowly allows your body to better adapt to new physical demands and prevents the discouragement that excessively sore muscles can cause.

EXPERIENCED   If you're already engaged in an exercise program, you may feel that you are capable of performing at the Experienced level. That's great. Just make sure to give yourself an honest assessment in each area: flexibility, strength (upper- and lower-body) and cardiovascular. For instance, if you're currently biking, swimming or jogging three times a week, you may be surprised by how challenging the flexibility or strength-training portions of the Fit in 15 program are. For these, you can perform at the Starter level while you perform at the Experienced level for the types of exercise your body is already well adapted to.

Sample Workout Program

This sample takes one of the options from each day of the week and compiles them into one full Fit in 15 workout program. Feel free to follow this program, or switch in one of the other workout options for that particular day listed in Part Three. Remember, there are several workouts to choose from in each section, and thousands of unique ways to combine these workouts into a program that's tailor-made for your needs, goals and experience level. You'll find overviews on the different types of fitness that make up the Fit in 15 program in the pages following this.

MONDAY Cardiovascular Training	Option 1: Brisk Walking (page 58) LEVEL: STARTER
TUESDAY Strength Training— Upper Body & Core	Option 3: Major Muscle Groups (pages 76–79) LEVEL: EXPERIENCED
WEDNESDAY Flexibility Training	Option 1: Standard Flexibility (pages 90–95) LEVEL: STARTER
THURSDAY Strength Training— Lower Body & Core	Option 3: Unilateral Moves (pages 118–21) LEVEL: STARTER
FRIDAY Cardiovascular Training	Option 4: Swimming (page 61) LEVEL: EXPERIENCED
SATURDAY Target Training	Option 2: Butt-Firming Workout (page 134) LEVEL: STARTER
SUNDAY Mind/Body Training	Option 3: Relax in a Hot Tub (page 140)

Cardiovascular Training

Cardiovascular training is perhaps the single most important type of training for your health since it works the most important muscle of your body—your heart. By elevating your heart rate, you increase the capacity of your heart to do work, and thereby strengthen it. A second benefit of cardiovascular exercise is that it encourages your body to burn energy (calories). When you ingest fewer calories than your body needs to maintain its weight, your body must turn to alternate sources of

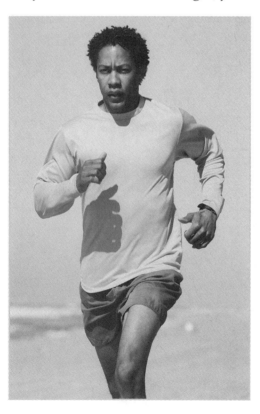

energy, and it often turns to stored body fat. Thus, by performing cardiovascular exercise and maintaining a reasonable diet, you are able to further improve your health and appearance.

While other types of training (such as training with weights) can be more effective at building muscle mass, cardiovascular exercise can also play a role. If you have been inactive, you will see improved muscle tone when you begin performing cardio work.

Finally, cardiovascular exercise will help you feel better and boost your energy levels by improving your body's efficiency. With more muscle and less body fat, it becomes easier to move. Cardiovascular training itself also helps you accommodate to moving, which is why a standard recommendation before going on an extended touring vacation is to begin walking on a regular basis for a month or two ahead of time—you don't want to feel out of shape or sluggish when you're supposed to be enjoying yourself! For all these reasons, cardiovascular training is one of the most important things you can do for your health, appearance and well-being.

Types of Cardiovascular Work

Essentially, any exercise that elevates your heart rate can be considered cardiovascular training. This might include walking, running, swimming, biking and the exercises performed on exercise equipment. Other types of exercise, such as flexibility training (yoga or Pilates) and strength training (both lower and upper body), have a cardiovascular component to them, but the aforementioned exercises are far better for cardiovascular health.

Heart Health

Life is full of ironies. Here is yet another: Cardiovascular training improves the health of your heart, but if you are unaccustomed to cardiovascular training, it can initially increase your risk of heart attack, especially if you are in an at-risk population. Those who have survived heart attacks begin a rehabilitation process that includes very carefully monitored cardiovascular exercise as a way to strengthen their hearts and lengthen their lives. This should indicate to you that cardiovascular exercise is good for everyone.

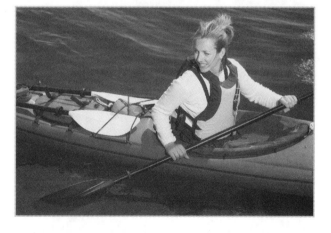

Rule number one of the cardiovascular program (and any exercise program) is to get your doctor's approval before you begin. With your doctor's blessing, you can begin training at a level that you feel comfortable with. Always begin more slowly rather than too quickly. You can always add more intensity or more time to cardiovascular work as you make improvements. While fat burning is correlated to how intensely you're working, you should strive to work within a range that's appropriate for your age and fitness level. This will assure the most fat-burning effect with the least amount of risk.

Cardiovascular work is safer if you slowly elevate your heart rate to your target zone. Then, at the end of your cardiovascular training, you should allow your heart rate to decelerate slowly. Spend the first couple of minutes and the last couple of minutes of each cardio training session working with less intensity than you do during the middle portion.

Cardio Equipment

SHOES

It goes without saying that you need shoes for outdoor walking or running, but walking, running and your favorite leisure activity each require a pair of shoes that's 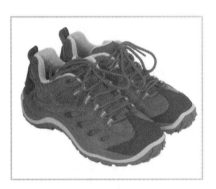 appropriate for that activity, especially if you're going to engage in this activity regularly. One of the single most common forms of injuries comes from wearing inappropriate footwear for these repetitive-motion exercises. If you plan to run, buy a good pair of running shoes. If you plan to walk, buy a good pair of walking shoes. A generic pair of "tennis shoes" is not always the best choice since these activities place stress on your hips, knees, ankles, feet and lower back. By choosing a pair of shoes that's suited for you and your activity, you will dramatically reduce the potential for injury.

It's also important to replace your training shoes often. While your shoes may still look almost new, after six months of use they may have lost much of the support that made them effective when you bought them. To be safe, buy new shoes sooner rather than later if you're using them regularly for exercise.

BICYCLES, TREADMILLS AND OTHER KINDS OF CARDIO EQUIPMENT

If you're plan is to be a casual bike rider, then almost any available bike will do. But if you want to be a more frequent bicyclist, then you may want to visit your local bike store and find a bike that's suitable for you and the kind of riding you intend to do. Other types of cardio equipment range from inexpensive (often mechanical) to very expensive (electrical), and includes stair steppers, treadmills, upright and recumbent bicycles, elliptical trainers and rowing machines. Many people belong to gyms so that they can use this equipment; others prefer to invest in a nice treadmill or stationary bike for their home. If you'd like to buy a piece of cardio equipment, make certain that you will enjoy and use it. Consider getting a short-term pass to a gym and training on the various types of equipment they have to help you with your decision.

SWIM GEAR

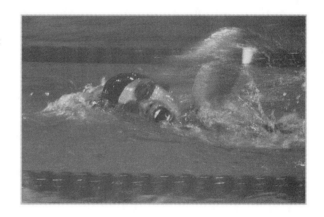

In addition to wearing swimwear that's appropriate and comfortable for swimming, you might also consider buying equipment to assist you in swimming: goggles help you see better and protect your eyes from chlorine in swimming pools; fins enable you to swim more powerfully by giving you more "kick." Perhaps one of the most useful pieces of swimming gear is a paddle board, a small flotation device that helps support some or all of your body weight to allow you to travel through the water more easily. These boards can also support your lower back if your midsection arches too much as you move through the water.

HEART-RATE MONITOR

Not only should you have the approval of a doctor to perform cardiovascular exercise, you should also consider buying a monitor to keep track of your heart rate. You can wear your heart-rate monitor while you exercise (unless you're in the water, of course) so that you get constant feedback about how your heart is responding to your exercise. Talk to your doctor to learn more about what is an appropriate exercising heart rate for you.

Strength Training

General fitness cardio and weight training are probably the two most popular forms of exercise that people perform primarily for their health benefits. Leisure activities such as tennis and golf, for instance, are also quite popular, but those who engage in them tend to do so more because the activities are enjoyable in and of themselves. Weight training, or strength training, is an important component of the Fit in 15 program. We've split strength training into two different workouts—upper-body training on Tuesdays and lower-body training on Thursdays. On each of these days, you'll often perform core work as well, which is discussed in the following section.

The most obvious benefit of strength training is increased muscle mass. Both men and women desire a little more muscle mass because they know that it gives them a healthier and more attractive appearance. Modest increases in muscle mass can also help your clothes fit better (or at the very least help you look better when you wear them). But, as important as this is, the most important fitness benefit of increased muscle mass is its effect on your metabolic rate. Muscle mass requires calories—the more muscle mass you have, the more calories you must consume each day just to maintain your weight. And, for the most part, the more calories your body needs to sustain itself, the less likely you are to increase your body fat stores. In addition to this huge perk, muscle mass gives you more padding and helps stabilize your skeleton, protecting you against injury. It also helps you overcome or ward off illness. Thus, the more muscle mass you have, the better.

Too Much Muscle?

Many people, particularly women, worry about getting so muscle bound that it makes them bulky. Please take this leap of faith: You won't get too muscular on this or almost any other muscle-building program. Thinking that you're working out so much that you'll get too muscular is a little like worrying that you'll get too rich if you work hard. Muscle mass is hard to add and if at first you feel you're getting too big, it is most likely because you're adding muscle mass faster than you're shedding body fat. Don't reduce your strength training—give the program a chance to work. Ultimately, the results of adding lean mass will have a slimming effect on your entire physique.

The Strength-Training Program

UPPER-BODY STRENGTH TRAINING   The muscles of the chest, shoulders, back and arms make up the upper body; training each of these groups is critical for men and women alike. A number of fitness programs that rely on cardiovascular exercises such as walking or jogging overlook the importance of upper-body strength. People who are weak in the upper body begin to have difficulty performing basic tasks such

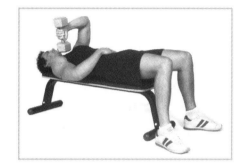

as carrying groceries or doing simple household chores as they age. Keeping your upper body strong is a key component of total-body fitness for now and for the rest of your life.

On Tuesdays, you will have five upper-body strength-training options. These workouts are all comparable and can be used interchangeably. Many have similar exercises, but all have a unique element. Read through the brief overviews to select the one or ones that appeal most to you. Regardless of the upper-body workout you choose, rest assured that you're balancing your body, building muscle mass and enhancing your appearance and longevity.

LOWER-BODY STRENGTH TRAINING   Thursdays offer you five lower-body strength workouts. Although other types of Fit in 15 workouts also target the lower body to some degree (cardiovascular and flexibility training, for instance, both use the muscles of the lower body, too), none of them targets muscle growth as effectively as strength training does. That's why it's important to devote one day a week of your program to lower-body training. You will not only add muscle mass, you will become stronger for other activities as well as better proportioned.

The lower body comprises multiple muscle groups, including the quads, hamstrings, calves and even glutes. Feel free to perform the workout program that appeals to you the most, but also recognize that switching programs from one week to the next may give you even better lower-body strength results.

WEIGHT SELECTION   The amount of weight you should use for your strength-training exercises depends on a number of variables, including the equipment you have available, your skill level and goals.

Availability: If you're only going to buy one set of dumbbells for all your exercises, choose a weight that's light enough for you to perform all the exercises in your program. This may mean a weight in the one- to three-pound range. To make a bigger financial investment in your training program, consider buying more than one pair of dumbbells (for instance, a set of three-, five- and ten-pounders). Or you might want to buy a pair of adjustable dumbbells; it can be a little time consuming changing from one weight to another, but this will give you flexibility in the amount of weight you can use for various exercises without having to purchase numerous sets of dumbbells.

Skill level: Starters should err on the side of a too-light weight rather than one that is too heavy. Ultimately, a workout regimen is one of the best ways to guard your body against injuries, but when you place new demands on your body, you are also more likely to injure yourself. By starting with lighter weights, you will reduce the potential for injury. Start slowly, and add more weight to your strength exercises as your body adapts. Starters should never feel that the weight is so heavy that they cannot complete the prescribed number of reps for any given exercise. If you find a particular move too challenging even with a one-pound weight, then attempt it with no weight; you can also hold a tennis ball or hand towel in your fist to better simulate the experience of lifting a weight.

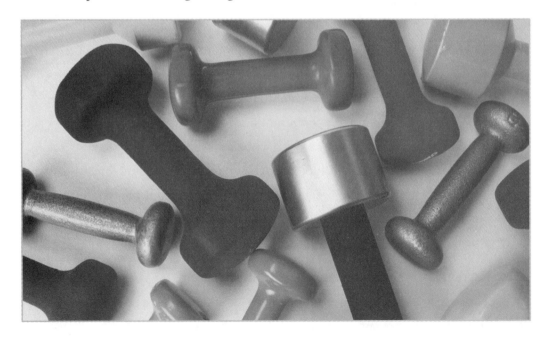

SELECTING THE RIGHT WEIGHT

LEVEL	APPROPRIATE WEIGHT
STARTER	Choose a weight that allows you to complete all the reps for every set of each exercise—this weight should not be the limiting factor for you. Sometimes you may not be able to perform every rep of every set based on pre-set conditions such as injury or a lack of conditioning following a period of inactivity, and that's fine. Work without weights for some exercises until you can perform all the reps.
EXPERIENCED Toning	Choose a weight that allows you to feel a burn in your target muscle when you're performing the set. You should be able to complete every rep of every set, allowing a short rest of 30-45 seconds between sets. If you're unable to finish each rep for a particular exercise, reduce the amount of weight for that exercise.
EXPERIENCED Muscle-building	Choose a weight that allows you to feel a significant burn and pumping sensation in your target muscle when you're performing the set. You may find that you cannot complete as many reps for your second or third sets as you could for your first set. As long as you can complete the target reps for your first set, you are using an appropriate weight. Those who are interested in building muscle can extend rest time to 45–60 seconds between sets for the same exercise.

Your goals: The more weight you use, the more muscular stimulation you provide your body and the more likely you are to increase your muscle mass. If your goal is toning your body rather than adding muscle mass, perform more repetitions with a lower weight. If your goal is building more muscle mass, use more weight and perform fewer reps. Use the guide above to select the weight that's right for you.

Good Form and Rep Pace

Many people think of weight training as something to be endured while they watch TV or listen to music, but you'll get much better results if you pay attention to what you're doing. Consider the following suggestions as you perform your Tuesday and Thursday strength-training workouts.

ALWAYS USE GOOD FORM.   Sloppy form often results from using a weight that is too light or too heavy so be sure to choose the right weight. Read the exercise instructions carefully—and re-read them frequently (if you return to the instructions after a couple months, you may be surprised to see how many elements of the move you've been neglecting or not performing correctly). Think of your workout technique as an art form and strive to perfect it. In essence, this means using your target muscle without relying too much on assisting muscles. Recruiting other muscles works against your purpose of developing all your muscle groups equally. Make certain that you focus on the muscle that the exercise targets.

CONTRACT YOUR MUSCLES AT THE TOP.   In the exercise descriptions, you are often instructed to isometrically contract your muscle (it won't happen just because you lift the weight) at the midway point of each rep. This additional squeeze increases the intensity and effectiveness of the exercise.

STRETCH THE MUSCLE AS YOU FINISH EACH REP.   In almost every exercise description is the instruction to stretch the muscle. Again, it's easy to avoid doing this since

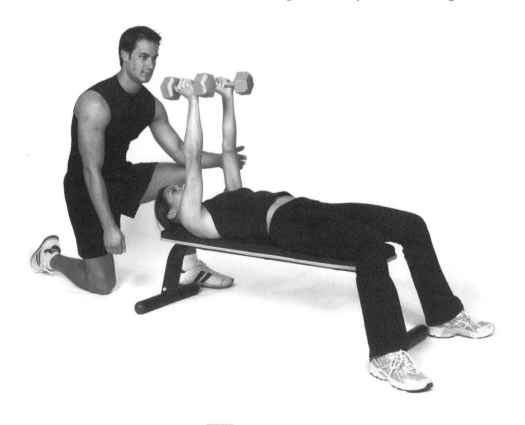

gravity will simply return the weight to its starting point without requiring much muscular effort from the exerciser. But this is ineffective: Muscles grow when they are stretched and contracted. Feeling the stretch in your target muscle is the second component of a well-executed repetition.

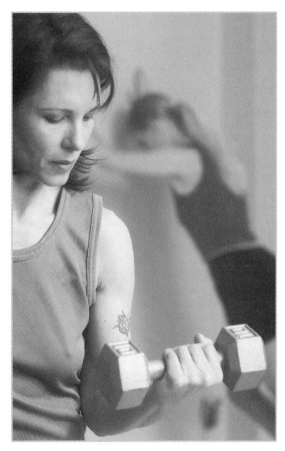

USE A SLOW TO MODERATE REP PACE. The speed at which you perform each rep may vary from person to person, but, in general, avoid speed work, where you perform reps quickly in a jerky fashion. This is far more likely to encourage injury than muscle building. As a base-line recommendation, it should take you about two seconds to perform the contracting phase of a rep and up to three seconds to perform the stretching phase. This is fairly slow, and most people will tend to work a little more quickly than this. That's fine, as long as you get that good contraction and stretch in each rep you perform.

REST AS MUCH AS YOU NEED TO BETWEEN SETS. These workouts are designed to be completed in about 15 minutes. Depending on many factors, especially on how long you rest between sets, the actual length of your workout may vary significantly. Determine whether your goal is to complete the workout as prescribed or to work out for only the allotted 15 minutes.

If you are a Starter, make sure that you are not elevating your heart too much (see page 20 for information on monitoring your heart rate) by working with too little rest. You may need to take up to a minute between sets, especially at the outset of your Fit in 15 program. Experienced trainers may also need to take time, especially if they are working to muscular fatigue in individual sets.

Keep in mind that you can perform these strength workouts in a "circuit," doing one set of each exercise before repeating a second set of any exercise. Alternatively, you may also perform all the sets for one exercise before moving on to the second exercise. The first option tends to increase the heart rate a bit more, boosting cardiovascular training and encouraging muscle toning. The second option tends to promote a little more muscle building as you effectively take each body part to a level of exhaustion before moving on to the next exercise and muscle group. Choose the strategy that best suits your goal and lifestyle.

Equipment

Buying all of the following equipment may be a terrific way to demonstrate your commitment to an exercise program, but it could also simply demonstrate your commitment to shopping. We recommend that you start slowly by buying a set of dumbbells, and then acquire more fitness equipment as your skills improve.

DUMBBELLS

A set of dumbbells is the single greatest need for a person beginning the Fit in 15 workout program. To get started, visit your local sports equipment store and select an appropriate set or sets of weights. (For more on this, see "Weight Selection" on page 31).

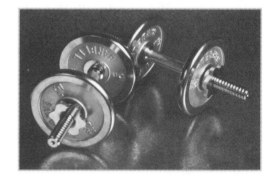

WEIGHT BENCH

A weight bench can be a very effective piece of equipment for completing many of the exercises included in the strength-training workouts. You can purchase a flat exercise bench or, better still, an adjustable one that allows for various incline angles. Regardless, make sure to buy a sturdy and stable bench—a number of less expensive models can be wobbly and dangerous, especially as they get older.

STABILITY BALL

Instead of—or in addition to—purchasing a weight bench, you can buy a stability
ball. These are far less stable than weight benches, but in this case that's a plus:

When you learn to perform the exercises on a
stability ball, you will also be training many
core muscles that support the larger muscles
targeted by the strength workouts. Stability
balls tend to be less expensive than weight
benches, but weight benches may be better for
Starters. Choose whichever you think best
serves your needs.

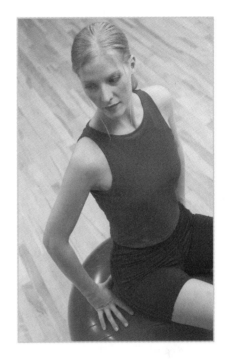

MOUNTED BAR FOR PULL-UPS

If you train at a gym, some form of pull-up bar
will likely be available to you. If you're working
out at home, you may have to buy and install
one. Try the type that fits into a doorway
(often, you can remove the bar from the
mounts when you finish your workouts). I recommend this optional piece of equipment because it is otherwise somewhat challenging to train your back muscles when
you're working out at home.

YOGA BLOCK

These lightweight yet durable and versatile foam blocks are a good choice for standing calf exercises, as well as some flexibility and balance moves. Yoga blocks are
lightweight and versatile.

Core Training

The abdominals are a relatively small muscle group composed of the abdominis rectus, obliques, serratus and intercostals, as well as a number of minor stabilizers that attach throughout the center of your body, but they sure do get a lot of attention. After winning the lottery, probably the next most popular selfish wish that people have is for a great six pack (or other improved body part). While winning the lottery is beyond your control, improving the look of your midsection (or "core") is possible through effort and dedication.

Having a strong core is not just a matter of vanity—it's crucial for fitness and health, and essential for strength, balance and cardiovascular training. A weak core will not provide you with enough stability to perform lower- and upper-body strength moves, and will thus also impede your ability to increase muscle mass. In addition, a weak core may lead to injury if your other muscle groups are comparatively stronger. For this reason, the Fit in 15 program groups core training with both upper- and lower-body strength training on Tuesdays and Thursdays. If your primary goal is a strong and sexy midsection, you can also do the Abs-Developing Workout on Saturday (see page 136).

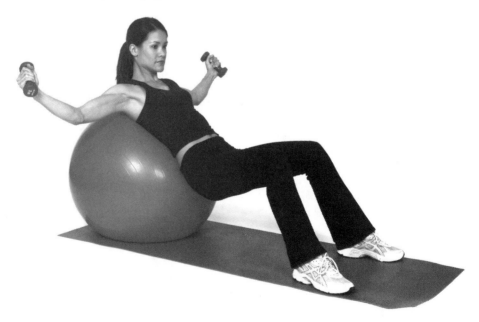

Get Your Abs On

Two essential elements in attaining attractive abs are: 1) having a small enough amount of body fat in your abdominal region so that the lines of your abs can be seen through the skin; 2) having enough muscular development of the abdominal region so that the lines are actually there to be viewed.

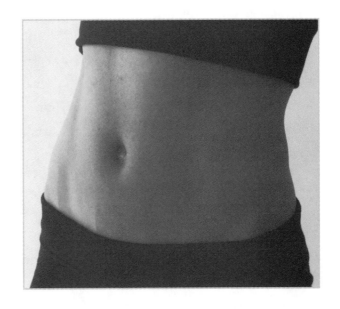

To achieve both of these, you must train your body for each of these goals. To reduce body fat, reduce caloric intake and increase calorie burning through cardiovascular and anaerobic (primarily weight-training) exercises.

Contradictorily, performing core movements is not the best way to burn the body fat from your abdominal region; these moves take relatively few calories to perform, making them an inefficient fat-burning choice of exercise.

However, core exercise is crucial for developing the lines and muscular detail of your midsection. To achieve truly impressive abdominals, you must work your core—and work it effectively. The rest of your program (diet, cardiovascular work and strength training) will then help make them visible for the world to see.

Making Your Abs Work for You

When it comes to core training, quality is far more important than quantity. The next time someone tells you that they perform hundreds of reps for core exercises every time they train, snicker to yourself—they're wasting their time and probably aren't getting very good results. (Still, this is better than no core work, unless it causes injury.) So how do you develop great core definition?

Here's the secret: Contract your abs as hard as you can on every rep you perform. Here's the second secret: Hold that contraction as you stretch back down to the starting position.

If you do both of these things, you won't be able to do very many reps before your abs reach exhaustion for that set. But this will work them much more effectively than performing dozens and dozens of wimpy reps.

The core exercises in Part Three include specific instruction on when and how to contract and stretch your abs. At first, this may prove challenging: if your core is weak or the moves are unfamiliar, you may not feel much of a contraction. But slowly and steadily, you will learn what this contraction means and how to use it to develop the midsection you want.

Core Training Parameters

Core moves are performed more than one day a week in the Fit in 15 program. Since core muscles are smaller muscles, they reach exhaustion quickly. However,

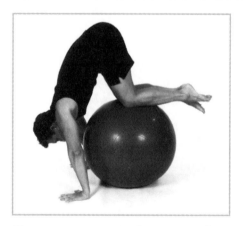

they also recover relatively quickly, allowing you to train them more frequently for better results. Still, you don't want to train your core every day. As with all muscle groups, they improve (both in terms of appearance and strength) from recovery.

In essence, the more frequently you recover fully from training them, the more effectively you will be in training your core.

If you were to train them every day, you simply wouldn't be able to get adequate recovery. That's why Fit in 15 recommends two days with core training, and a potential third target day if that's one of your primary goals. Two to three days of core training is ideal for exercisers of all skill levels.

REP COUNTS

Many people train their midsections with far too many sets and reps. This leads to "sparing" the amount of work your body has to do for each single rep, undercutting the total benefit of the program. In the Fit in 15 workout, the rep recommendations per set vary typically vary from 10 to 15, no matter your skill level. As you get more comfortable with the program, you may feel sometimes that 15 reps is just too easy.

When this happens, it means you aren't working hard enough for each rep. Force yourself to bring more intensity to each rep. Don't conserve your energy, work harder! Here are some tips to make each rep count:

1) Slow down your rep pace. Instead of taking 2–3 seconds per rep, start taking 5–10 seconds.

2) Contract harder when you get to the top of the movement for each rep.

3) Try a double contraction at the top of each rep. Squeeze down once then, without releasing, squeeze down again. Now that's tough!

4) Really hold that contraction tight as you stretch back down to finish your rep.

5) Don't release your abs between reps. Hold your abs tight as you transition into the next rep.

Try all these intensity techniques as your skill level increases and learn to work to muscular fatigue with 15 or fewer reps.

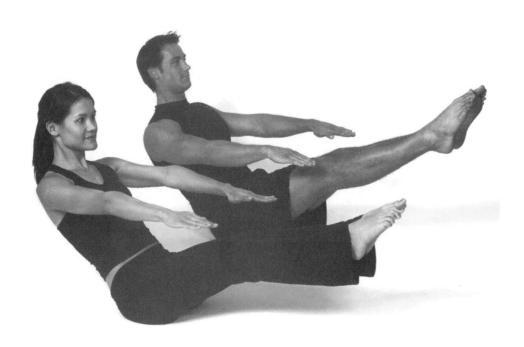

Different Targets

Crunches on the ball are one of the all-time great exercises for developing a well-defined and strong core, but if they're the only move you're using, then you aren't fully training your abs. Make sure to include a variety of exercises in your core training. The Fit in 15 program contains several core movements, each targeting your midsection in a slightly different way—make good use of this variety in your personalized program.

Equipment

While you don't need any equipment to perform the floor moves, you may find the following useful:

STABILITY BALL

We use an exercise ball in some of the core moves. While you can make exercise substitutions rather than using a ball, I highly recommend an exercise ball because it is versatile for other exercises, too. Abs crunches done on a ball is one of the most effective and easiest-to-perform moves for improving the strength and appearance of your midsection.

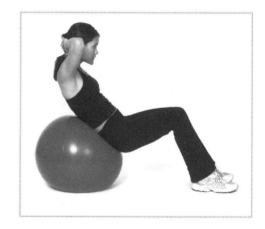

MAT

A yoga mat is versatile, and though many are not very thick, they provide a nice non-slip cushion for your body, especially your tailbone.

Flexibility Training

As we age, our muscles lose pliability and certain movements become more challenging. By incorporating flexibility training into your weekly training program, you will not only be able to maintain your range of motion, you'll actually be able to improve it, especially with regard to areas that you have neglected.

Flexibility training tends to be a love it/hate it endeavor. Most people who exercise either include it in almost every workout (such as those devoted to Pilates, yoga or tai chi) or barely do it at all (those who tend to rely on muscle-building or cardiovascular exercise). While it's a fine idea to include flexibility work on a daily basis, you don't want to perform *only* flexibility work. Include other types of training to be fully fit.

On the flip side, if you are inclined not to do it at all, start incorporating flexibility moves regularly in your training. The Fit in 15 program sets aside one day a week for you to focus exclusively on flexibility training. Feel free to add these moves to your other workout days as part of your warm-up or cool-down, and consider adding a second day of flexibility training as your target-training option on Saturdays.

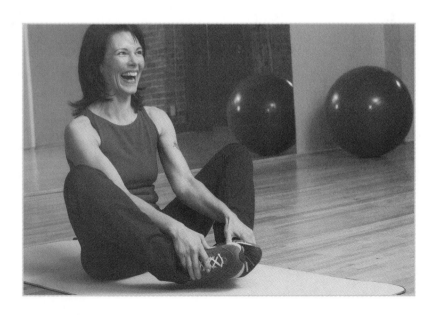

Types of Stretching

You've probably heard that the best way to perform flexibility work is to "stretch and hold," where you maintain a flexibility posture for 30 or so seconds. While this is certainly an excellent strategy, the Fit in 15 program also increases flexibility

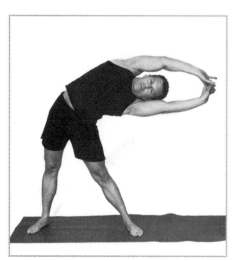

using movement. Moving gently from one flexibility position to another creates more body heat, allowing your muscles to become more pliable. This gentle movement can often help you achieve a deeper stretch than the more static version.

A third option is the ballistic type of stretching, where you move aggressively into stretch poses. This is a good technique for those who need to develop sudden bursts of energy in stretch positions (such as

gymnasts), but because of the increased chance of injury associated with this type of stretching, the Fit in 15 program emphasizes slow, static stretches and gentle movement stretches.

Risks of Flexibility Training

As with cardiovascular training, assess the gains and risks of flexibility training before beginning a training regimen. If you have not stretched much recently, you run the risk of injury when you first start a stretching program, especially if you notice that you are particularly stiff in one place or if you have a recurring injury.

Before you begin a flexibility training regimen, you should get your doctor's permission. After that, you might also consider seeking a qualified expert to assess the kind of program that's best for you. Your doctor, a physical therapist, a qualified personal trainer, a yoga teacher or Pilates instructor—anyone who can offer one-on-one corrections—is an excellent option for helping you to make the most of your flexibility while reducing the risk of injury.

Equipment

You could perform stretching workouts without any equipment, but the following pieces of equipment may be beneficial for helping you maintain better postures while stretching, and thus allow you to gain more from your flexibility training.

MAT

A mat provides comfort and support, espe-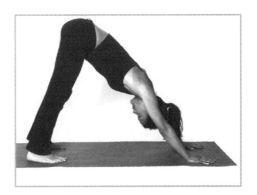
cially for movement sequences such as the
Down Dog series. On a wood floor, a yoga
mat will give you a bit of padding to
remove some pressure from your hands,
feet and, occasionally, knees. Using the mat
on carpet helps prevent slipping. This is the
top equipment recommendation for improv-
ing your flexibility training. You can also use your mat for your core training and
during many of your strength-training exercises.

YOGA BLOCK

Yoga blocks can help adjust one body part compared to another. For instance, by placing a block (or a folded blanket) under your butt while performing the seated straddle stretch, you may be able to increase the amount of the stretch or the duration for which you can hold it.

BROOMSTICK, TOWEL OR STRAP

Any of these can be used to help support upper-body flexibility training. For instance, holding a broomstick, towel or strap in your hands overhead as you perform a side stretch can help you open your shoulders, elongate your spine and, ultimately, deepen your side stretch. A strap is also beneficial for assisting with hamstrings stretches and other moves; you can place the strap around your foot and gently hold it, allowing you to deepen the stretch.

Target Training

Target training allows you to really personalize your Fit in 15 program. Each Saturday, you will perform a workout that emphasizes your primary goal. This goal can be the same as one of the workouts for the other days of the week—for instance, you may want to do more cardio, flexibility or upper-body and core training in your program. If that's the case, then simply add another workout from one of those days, or even repeat the workout you performed earlier in the week.

However, many people will have a goal that requires a workout that's slightly different than those of the previous training days. For example, you may have started the Fit in 15 program to firm up your butt, tighten your thighs, build upper-body muscle or develop your abs. If one of these goals is your target, then you can simply follow the extra workout that addresses your specific target-training goal.

Determine Your Target-Training Goal

Many people already have a clear idea of their target-training goal. If you don't have one yet, then you should think about it as you begin your Fit in 15 program. First, are you more interested in anaerobic (muscle-building) or aerobic (cardiovascular) training? What do you consider your greatest fitness weakness? Is it upper-body

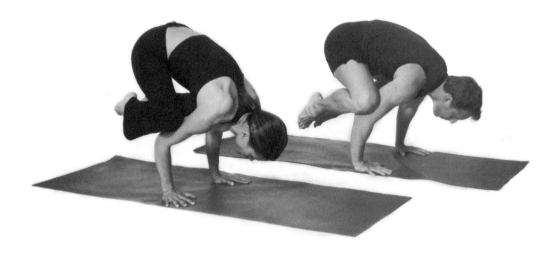

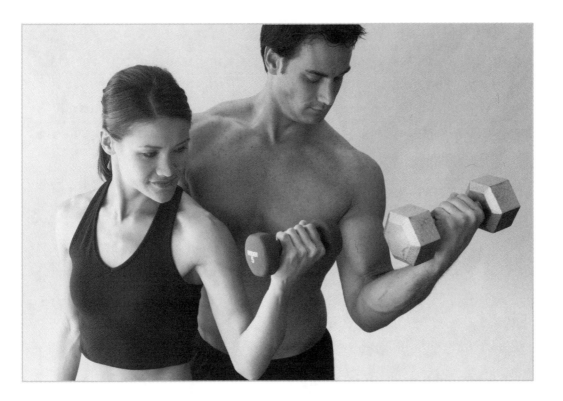

strength? A midsection or lower body that you'd like to tone and define? The answer to these questions will help you determine your target-training goal.

Below are several target-training descriptions. Read through them, select your target-training goal, then turn to Part Three to find the appropriate workout.

ARM-TONING

Many people, especially women, want to emphasize toning their arms. Recently, triceps were the muscles of the moment in Hollywood, with every actress in town pursuing the attractive indentation at the back of the arm. The arm-toning workout in Part Three will help you develop this indentation as well as gain more tone and definition for your whole arm.

BUTT-FIRMING

While the Tuesday lower-body-and-core workout targets your whole legs, this target-training workout really works the butt. Its a great complement to the lower-body workout, giving your backside a double dose of toning each week.

THIGH-TIGHTENING

Perhaps your biggest problem area is your thighs rather than your whole lower body. If this is the case, consider using the Thigh-Tightening Workout on Saturdays as a complement to your lower-body-and-core workout on Thursdays. Strength training your lower body twice a week will have a dramatic effect on your muscle tone and definition.

TOTAL BODY FAT–REDUCING

This weight training–based workout will greatly support your twice-weekly cardio-vascular workouts in reducing body fat. For this workout, you will alternate between upper- and lower-body weight-training exercises, trying to keep moving throughout your 15-minute workout. Performing anaerobic work such as weight lifting in a continuous fashion increases your heart rate and your body fat–burning capacity, as well as improves the muscle tone of your entire body.

UPPER-BODY MUSCLE-BUILDING

Many people choose an exercise program that relies almost entirely on upper-body weight training. Since Fit in 15's well-rounded fitness program is based on many different types of fitness, you may feel that you want to perform more upper-body muscle building than the program otherwise includes. The workout in Part Three relies on the best muscle-building exercises for the largest upper body muscle groups (chest, back and shoulders), and emphasizes performing more sets for each exercise to better stimulate muscle growth.

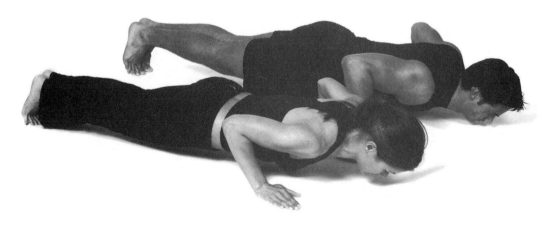

ABS-DEVELOPING

As mentioned in the Core Training section, there are two steps in building great abs: learning to work your abs effectively to define them, and following a proper nutrition program to allow for a low enough level of body fat that your abs are visible through your skin. The basic Fit in 15 program includes core work on both Tuesdays and Thursdays, but if you really want to develop appealing abs, you can also include a full workout of just abs exercises. The workout in Part Three gives you a 15-minutes abs routine you can perform as your Saturday target-training workout.

FLEXIBILITY-ENHANCING

If flexibility is your primary concern, then consider a second day of flexibility training during your Saturday target-training workout. Perform one of the workouts

listed in the Wednesday Flexibility Training chapter or attend a yoga class (this can also be considered additional mind/body training, as yoga is an option for that). Keep in mind that gym or studio yoga classes always run longer than 15 minutes (a half hour is often the minimum; they're generally 90 minutes). Still, if you have time in your schedule, performing an hour to an hour and a half of yoga once

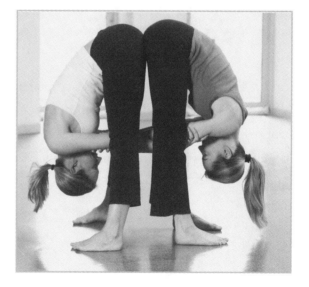

a week is an excellent complement to your other Fit in 15 training. For other specific flexibility workouts, see Wednesday workouts starting on page 88.

CARDIO-ENHANCING

If your target-training goal is to improve your cardiovascular health or to reduce body fat levels (or both), then opt to perform a third day of cardiovascular training a week by adding a session of cardiovascular work to your target-training Saturday. You can repeat one of the workouts you're already doing, or add in a new type of

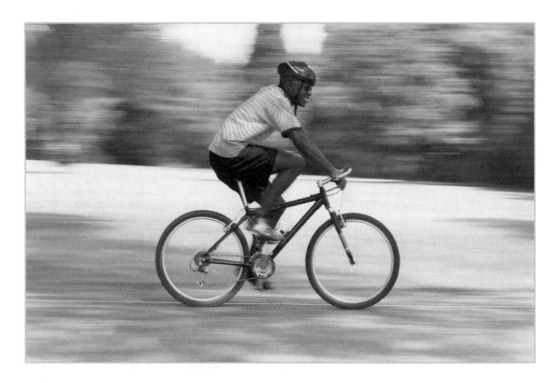

cardio training. While it's perfectly acceptable to do the same cardio workout three times a week, you might gain even more benefit from trying a different type of workout. Consider adding a bike ride or a swim if you're not already doing these activities. For other specific cardiovascular workouts, see Cardio Workouts starting on page 56.

Mind/Body Training

The average American lifestyle is very hectic, with all cylinders running from the moment you get up in the morning. This may carry you through most of the day as you deal with the responsibilities of work, school and family, but by the end of the

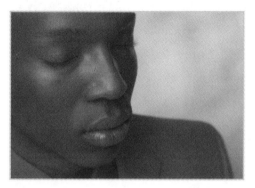

day, you may feel exhausted and barely able to think, let alone move effectively.

A constant bombardment of stress hormones such as cortisol greatly increases your chances of developing illnesses such as cancer or heart disease. However, taking a few minutes once a week (or a few times a week) to reduce the stimulation of your brain can have a dramatic impact on the chemicals within your body and increase your long-term health and well-being. The only time many of us shut down our focus on our busy lives is when we stop to watch TV or sleep, but neither activity fully lets you be introspective.

Perform mind/body training at least once a week to allow your body time to repair itself. Set aside 15 or more quiet minutes to think about how the sensation of relaxation feels. Mind/body training can also include participating in any activity that generates a peaceful feeling and releases endorphins. Almost everything we do in life is stressful, and finding a way to combat the ravaging effects of stress is one of the best ways to enhance your longevity.

Mind/Body Activities

See which type of mind/body activity appeals most to you:

MASSAGE

Massage is the classic way to relieve stress and sore muscles, and it can be any length of time, from a short chair massage, to one at your doctor's office, to a full-

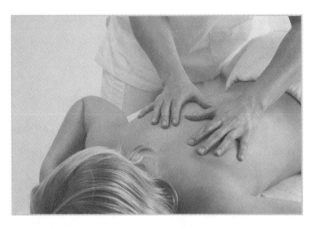

day treatment at a spa. While the Fit in 15 program emphasizes short workouts in general, feel free to indulge with a full-hour massage or longer. Initially, getting a massage may almost seem like a workout (you might have some tight spots or knots that are a little painful when massaged); the release of tension even causes your body to repair itself in a way that's similar to how your body responds to exercise. As your body adapts to massage, however, it becomes even more relaxing.

One of the keys to a good massage is finding the masseuse that's right for you. Ask friends and relatives for recommendations, or seek out a certified masseuse from a spa or doctor's office. During the massage, communicate to the masseuse if something hurts or if the masseuse is using too much or too little pressure.

WARM BATH

Water's restorative quality makes it easy to relax while soaking in water. Warm water can also help you overcome muscle soreness associated with other workouts in your Fit in 15 program. Taking a warm bath is one of the easiest and least expensive of the mind/body-training options. It's also something you can do more frequently than once a week. If at all possible, consider taking a relaxing bath two or three times a week, and engaging in some other mind/body activity for your Sunday workout. Feel free to add Epsom or other bath salts—or even bubbles—for their soothing and/or recovery-enhancing effects.

HOT TUB

Soaking in hot water can be restorative and relaxing, and it can also help you over-come muscle soreness associated with other workouts in your Fit in 15 program. The motion of the water in a hot tub can prove even more relaxing than the still water of your bathtub. If you don't have a hot tub in your home or apartment complex, try a spa and gym.

STEAM ROOM

The wet heat of a steam room can soothe your body and help you relax. Generally, steam rooms are considerably warmer than either hot tubs or baths. At first, you may find the temperature uncomfortable, and you will certainly find yourself sweating, but sweating helps your body purify itself of toxins. Steam rooms are also good for helping you reduce muscle soreness from your other Fit in 15 training days.

SLOW STRETCH

The Fit in 15 program already deems Wednesday your Flexibility Training day, but you can also consider adding a session of yoga, Pilates or slow stretches for your mind/body training on Sundays. While the purpose of the flexibility workouts is to help you improve your range of motion and muscular pliability, the purpose of the mind/body slow-stretch day is to allow you to relax and focus on the connection between your mental processes and the physical movement of your body. Yoga is particularly good for this: Many yoga instructors emphasize relaxation techniques and the mind/body connection over the exercise-related benefits of the movement, although you should check with the studio/gym and the instructor beforehand regarding the goal of the class. Often, yoga classes run much longer than 15 minutes, but many are available early in the morning for those who like to start their day with a stretch.

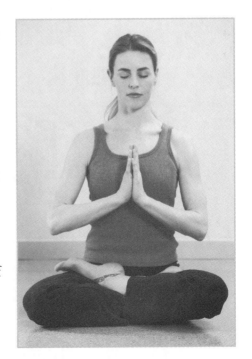

MEDITATION OR PRAYER

These introspective disciplines mean different things to different people, but often a spiritual connection to your thought processes can provide the same type of mind/body training that other forms of relaxation offer. If you find that meditation or prayer relaxes or rejuvenates you, then this may be a great mind/body-training option for you.

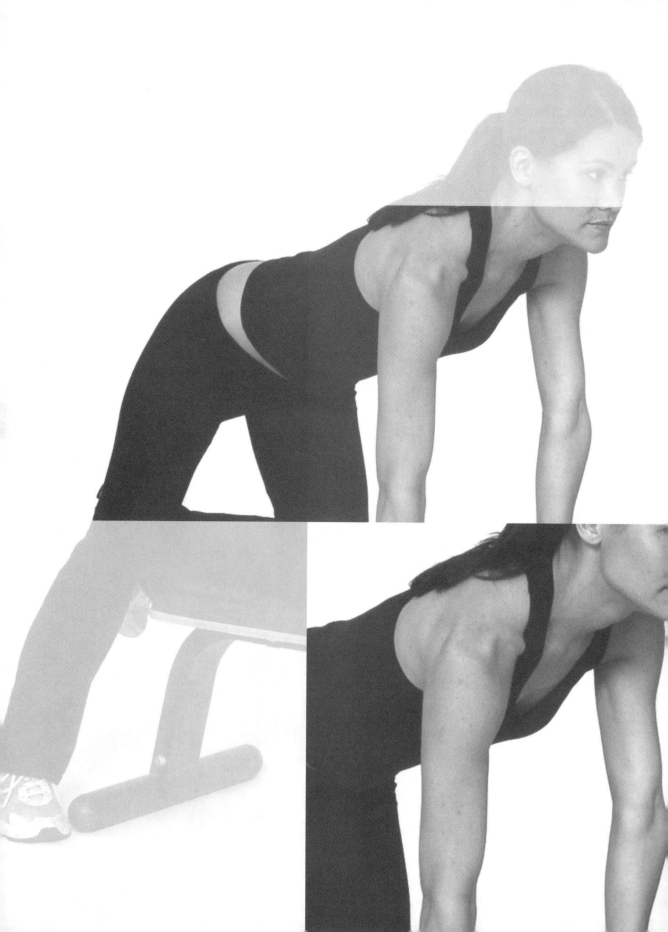

Part 3

workouts

Monday

cardio workouts

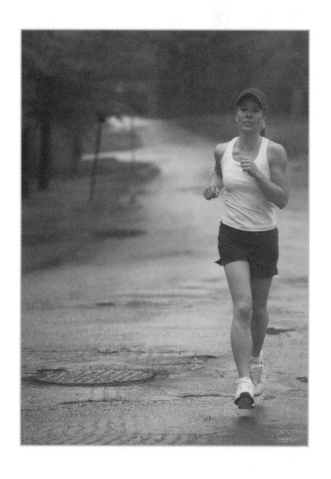

The Fit in 15 program offers eight different cardiovascular options to choose from for your Monday and Friday workouts. Select the form of training that appeals most to you. Here, we offer brisk walking, light jogging/running, bicycling, swimming, water walking or aerobics, treadmill, other cardio equipment and an easy-does-it walk.

Consider mixing up your workouts from one session to another. It's also a great idea to change the pace at which you work. Some days, you may have a lot of energy and might want to include a few minutes of light jogging with your brisk walk. On days when you're less energetic or you feel like you're still a little sore from the workouts of the previous days, you might consider an easy-does-it walk.

OPTION 1	Brisk Walking
OPTION 2	Light Jogging/Running
OPTION 3	Bicycling
OPTION 4	Swimming
OPTION 5	Water Walking/Aerobics
OPTION 6	Treadmill
OPTION 7	Other Exercise Equipment
OPTION 8	Easy-Does-It Walking

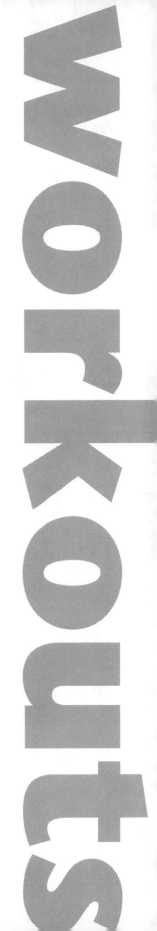

1. BRISK WALKING   LEVEL: STARTER/EXPERIENCED

One of the best and most effective forms of cardiovascular exercise is brisk walking. The goal is not to walk as fast as you can so much as it is to walk at a pace that allows your heart rate to elevate. If your breathing is too labored for conversation, reduce your walking pace. Working at this intensity level effectively exercises your heart and encourages fat burning.

HOW TO WALK

Start out more slowly than your peak rate, and gradually increase your speed so that your heart rate accelerates comfortably. As you walk, you can move your arms; this helps burn more calories while also toning your core muscles. A couple of minutes before you finish your 15-minute walk, drop your pace a bit so that your heart rate gradually diminishes. If you feel a tendency to "sprint" to the end of your walk, it's fine to do so, as long as you walk slowly for a couple of minutes afterwards to allow your heart rate to safely decelerate.

More experienced exercisers can accelerate and decelerate a little more quickly, spending more time overall at their peak heart rates.

WHERE TO WALK

You can do your brisk walk either indoors or outdoors. Walking outdoors is a great option if the climate permits—choose this option as often as you can. If working indoors, find a place where you can walk freely without having to adjust your pace for turns too frequently (malls and large public buildings are often good choices). You can also walk at a gym if it has a track. Keep in mind that small tracks can increase the amount of stress your lower body must absorb due to frequent turning (generally stressing one side more than the other). Often, these types of tracks will have traffic move one way some days of the week and the other direction on other days of the week. Try to alternate directions from one workout to the next.

2. LIGHT JOGGING/RUNNING   LEVEL: EXPERIENCED

A 15-minute jog or run can be a great way to start the day. Not only will you get your heart pumping, you'll also burn more calories than you will while walking at a brisk pace. Before you start a jogging or running program, talk to your doctor to make sure that it's a safe activity for you since both can have a profound effect on your heart rate.

HOW TO JOG/RUN

First, make sure you have top-quality running shoes in good condition. Running is stressful on the body, and good shoes are crucial in helping you prevent injury from impact. Start slowly, taking the first couple of minutes to warm up and gently allow your heart rate to accelerate. Then, for the next ten minutes or so, joggers should choose a pace that allows you to carry a conversation with someone; runners should run at a sustainable pace where you are breathing deeply but smoothly (you may or may not be able to carry on a sustained and comfortable conversation, but err on the side of safety). At the end of your jog/run, slow your pace for the last few minutes to allow your heart rate to gradually return to its resting rate. Runners can sprint to the end of their run, but remember to spend an extra minute or two moving (slow jog or brisk walk) to decelerate your heart rate.

To avoid injury, think about "gliding" as you connect with the ground for every stride, stepping lightly and pulling the weight of your body horizontally along the ground rather than landing vertically with all your weight on your leading leg. The best way to do this is to elongate your stride, even if it slows you down (this will also encouraging muscle building in your legs).

WHERE TO JOG/RUN

You can jog or run indoors or outdoors. If you do so indoors, you should probably seek out a gym or indoor track facility. Keep in mind that small tracks can increase the amount of stress your lower body must absorb due to frequent turning. Often, these types of tracks will have traffic move one way some days of the week and the other direction on other days of the week. Try alternate directions from one workout to the next.

When jogging or running outdoors, avoid cement. Initially, jogging on cement may cause you no problems, but since it doesn't absorb the weight of your body, your body must absorb the force of each impact, resulting in damage to knees and other body parts. The damage is cumulative but you may not notice until pain or injury seems to come on suddenly. Blacktop is a good option, but outdoor tracks and grassy areas (such as parks) are even better.

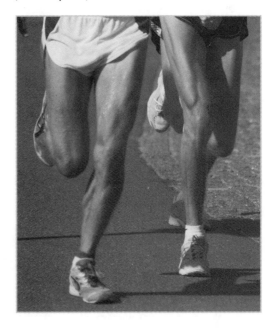

3. BICYCLING   LEVEL: STARTER/EXPERIENCED

Bicycle riding can be a great form of exercise for people of all experience levels. It's both a great Starter or Experienced way to get in your cardiovascular training. People in some parts of the country will find that bicycle riding, unfortunately, is a seasonal endeavor. If that's the case for you, then consider stationary biking as a substitute at other times of year. Either purchase a stationary bike for home, or join a gym where one is available.

HOW TO BIKE

This workout presumes that you have mastered the skill of riding a bike. Once you've done that, this activity can be as simple as a leisurely pedal through the neighborhood to an intense Lance Armstrong–like challenge. Regardless of your level, start slowly. For the first two or three minutes of your ride, pedal easily and fairly steadily, allowing your body to warm up and grow accustomed to

the activity. Starters can maintain this gentle pace throughout their entire ride. More Experienced riders can pick up the pace, pedaling steadily, allowing their heart rate to accelerate. When it comes to hills, you should feel a little bit of a burn in your legs as you pump your way up to the top. At the end of the ride, regardless of your level, make a concerted effort to reduce the intensity of your work for the last two or three minutes, allowing your heart rate to decelerate a bit before you stop. At the end of your ride, you can gently stretch for a minute or two to help reduce any fatigue or soreness that you might experience.

WHERE TO RIDE

Unless you live in a congested area, you can probably start your ride right from your home. If not, consider buying a bike rack for your car so that you can carry your bike to an appropriate place for bike riding.

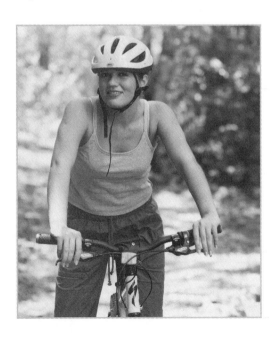

4. SWIMMING

LEVEL: STARTER/EXPERIENCED

Swimming is one of the most beneficial forms of exercise. It stimulates your cardiovascular system and also gives you a good anaerobic (muscle-building) workout. Each time you pull your arm through the water, it's similar to performing a repetition of a weight-training movement.

HOW TO SWIM

While teaching you specific swimming techniques is beyond the scope of the Fit in 15 program, we encourage you to seek out instruction if you are unfamiliar with swimming strokes and execution (many pools and gyms with pools offer swimming classes and instruction). If you're already familiar with swimming, then it's a great selection to include on your Cardiovascular Training days.

During your swim you can perform one stroke (such as American crawl, breast stroke or back stroke), or switch strokes after every few laps. As with other forms of cardio, start each session at a more leisurely pace, increase the pace for the bulk of the workout, and then work less strenuously at the end to allow your heart rate to gradually reduce. Regardless of whether you are a Starter or Experienced swimmer, this form of cardiovascular exercise is one of the best. Starters can take it easy, making their strokes more leisurely. Experienced swimmers can stroke more dynamically, raising their heart rate a little more.

WHERE TO SWIM

When swimming at public pools, follow all rules of etiquette, including using the appropriate lane or lanes for your skill level. Other swimmers tend to get a little hostile if you get over ambitious and jump into a lane that's beyond your skill level.

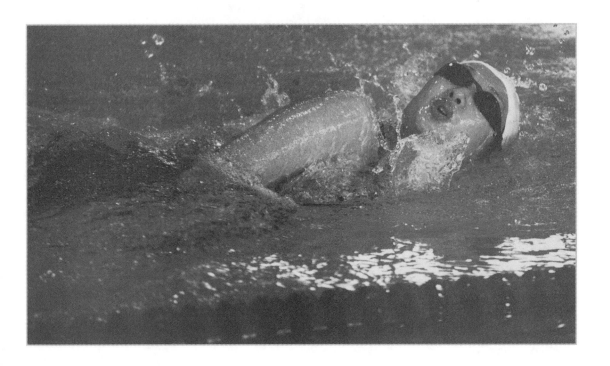

5. WATER WALKING/AEROBICS   LEVEL: STARTER

If you like the idea of a water workout but don't want to swim, you can also choose one of these water option: water walking or water aerobics.

WATER WALKING

Walking through water is very good cardiovascular and anaerobic (muscle-building) work. You might also be surprised at how challenging it is but adaptable to almost every skill level. That said, this form of exercise is better classified as Starter level rather than Experienced. First, find a pool where the lanes are of a consistent depth (usually three to four feet deep). When you walk from one end of the pool to the other, you'll begin to feel your heart rate accelerate, especially if you push your body through the water with much force. You'll also notice that it takes a lot of lower-body and core strength to move through the water.

WATER AEROBICS

Water aerobics are often taught at gyms that have a pool. While it's beyond the scope of the Fit in 15 program to give you detailed instruction on how to build your own water aerobics routine, consider joining a water aerobics class for a short period of time to learn the basic moves. Choose the ones that appeal to you the most and construct your own 15-minute water aerobics routine.

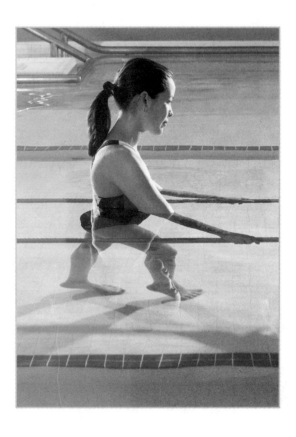

6. TREADMILL   LEVEL: STARTER/EXPERIENCED

The advice for working out on a treadmill is similar to that for leisurely walking, briskly walking, jogging or running, whichever activity you plan to do on a treadmill. Read through the descriptions of the pace that appeals to you the most to determine how to incorporate that pacing into your treadmill work.

In addition to the advice on pacing, adapt the following considerations into your treadmill training. First, pay attention to what you're doing! When you read or watch TV while on a treadmill (which many people do), you're more likely to lose your balance and tumble off the treadmill (which many people do). Especially at first, treadmills are trickier than regular stride movements on the ground because you don't receive the visual cues from movement—you're essentially staying in place while the equipment moves under you. Make use of your eyes and the handrails (if available) to help you get accustomed to the movement.

Use the incline button to change up your workout. Many treadmills can elevate to different levels. The steeper the incline, the more challenging the work and the more calories you are likely to burn. If you'd like, you can simply perform your treadmill work at a low incline (about 3 degrees), but you can also adjust it up to 7 or 10 or more degrees for more intense cardiovascular work. It's a good idea to change up the amount of incline so that you don't overwork your body at one angle—continually working at a set angle is more likely to cause a repetitive-motion type of injury than working at a variety of different angles. Consider changing your incline level every three minutes or so.

7. OTHER EXERCISE EQUIPMENT   LEVEL: STARTER/EXPERIENCED

Using cardio equipment is a great way to stay in shape during the winter when you can't get outside to exercise. Many people find they like exercise equipment so much that they prefer to use it year-round. People also tend to realize that they prefer one type of equipment over another. Here are some options:

STANDARD STEP MACHINES

With these machines, your weight sinks the step as you shift from one side to the other. By using the adjustable levels, you can make this an easy or challenging cardio workout.

STEP MILL MACHINES

These miniature escalators move in reverse: you climb the steps while the steps roll down. This is one of the most challenging forms of cardio equipment because you are constantly stepping upwards, moving your full body weight with each step. Adjustable levels affect the rate at which the stairs roll, allowing you to make this a very challenging workout (but, even on a low level, 15 minutes on a step mill is a challenging workout).

UPRIGHT BIKE MACHINES

Some find the seats on these standard machines a little uncomfortable, but they are probably a little more effective for fat burning than the recumbent variety since the recumbent version encourages you to relax.

RECUMBENT BIKE MACHINES

These are a little more comfortable than the upright bike version and are great for calorie burning. You can increase the resistance level of the pedals if you want to increase your work. You can set the program to a steady rate at whichever level you desire, or follow one of the preset programs built into the machine.

ELLIPTICAL TRAINER

These "gliding" machines are a great choice for those who want to avoid impact or repeated bending of the knees.

ROWING MACHINES

This is one of the few cardiovascular exercise machines that work the upper body, and is thus a good selection.

8. EASY-DOES-IT WALKING   LEVEL: STARTER/EXPERIENCED

A slow walk can be as beneficial as jogging and brisk walking. Some starters may feel much more comfortable performing a leisurely walk than any other type of cardiovascular work, especially for the first month or two of their program. Experienced trainers may find that on certain days, a leisurely walk sounds far more appealing than a strenuous jog or session on a piece of cardio equipment. Include this type of easier cardiovascular work on days when it's appropriate for you.

The recommendations for a leisurely walk are simple: Just go do it. Spend 15 minutes moving at any pace that is comfortable for you. Remember—easy does it.

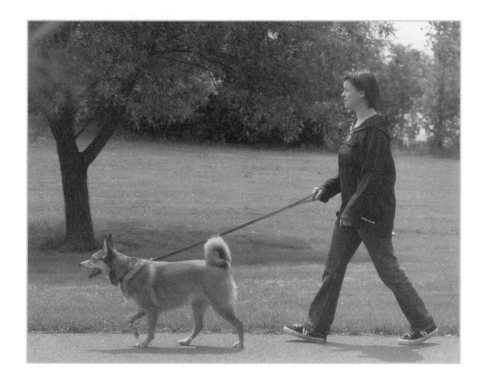

Tuesday

strength workouts— upper body & core

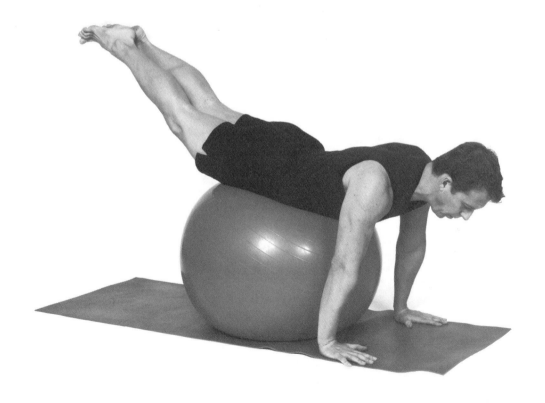

For your Tuesday workouts, you'll have five workout options to choose from. Each of these is an excellent upper body and core workout that you can complete in about 15 minutes. Choose the one that appeals to you most on any given Upper Body & Core training day. One week, you may feel like doing the optimal Primary Moves Workout. Another day you may feel more like using your body weight with Option 4. Perform whichever workout you want from this section on Tuesday. It's a great idea to switch from one workout to another from one week to the next, but you'll also get great results if you find that you like one workout better than the others and simply want to do that workout on most Tuesdays.

OPTION 1	Primary Moves
OPTION 2	Secondary Moves
OPTION 3	Major Muscle Groups
OPTION 4	Body Weight Moves
OPTION 5	Easy Does It

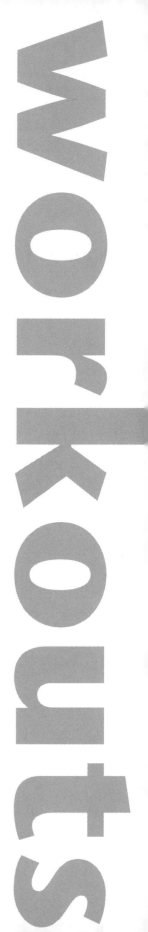

Tuesday option 1

Primary Moves

This Primary Moves option targets each of your upper body muscle groups, including chest, shoulders, back, triceps and biceps, as well as your core. It's a great total-body toner or muscle builder. Starters should perform two sets of each exercise while Experienced exercisers should perform three sets.

For more of a muscle-building emphasis, finish all sets of one exercise before moving on to the next exercise. For more of a toning emphasis, use the circuit-training technique where you complete one set of each exercise, and then go through the exercise list a second or third time, depending on your experience level (e.g., do one set of Chest Presses then one set of Overhead Shoulder Presses, one set of Dumbbell Rows, etc. Return to the top of the list again once you reach the bottom.)

EXERCISES	STARTER Sets/Reps	EXPERIENCED Sets/Reps
Chest Presses	2/10	3/12
Overhead Shoulder Presses	2/10	3/12
Dumbbell Rows	2/10	3/12
Triceps Extensions	2/10	3/12
Alternating Curls	2/10	3/12
Ball Crunches	2/10	3/12

CHEST PRESSES   TARGET: CHEST

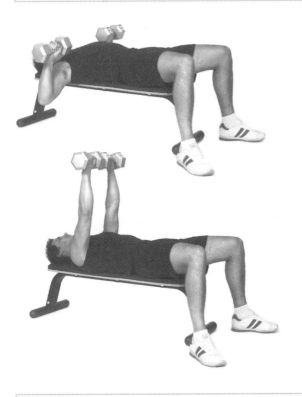

SETUP: Place the center of your back on a balance ball or lie on a flat weight bench. Hold a dumbbell in each hand near your armpits.

MOVEMENT: Use the strength of your chest to press the weights up until your arms are fully extended. Stop short of locking out your elbows and contract your chest muscles for a moment. Return to the starting position, concentrating on feeling a stretch across your chest.

OVERHEAD SHOULDER PRESSES   TARGET: SHOULDERS

SETUP: Sit on a balance ball or a weight bench (the bench can be flat, or upright for more back support). Hold a dumbbell in each hand with your elbows near your sides and your hands just above shoulder height.

MOVEMENT: Press the weights up until your arms are fully extended. Without locking out your shoulders or elbows, contract the muscles on the sides of your shoulders for a moment. Return to the starting position, concentrating on feeling a stretch in your shoulders.

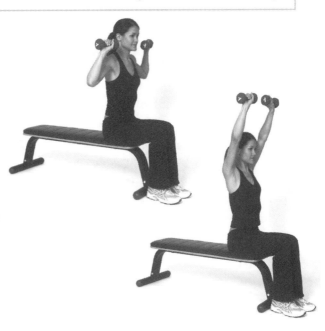

TUESDAY

Upper Body & Core

DUMBBELL ROWS

TARGET: BACK

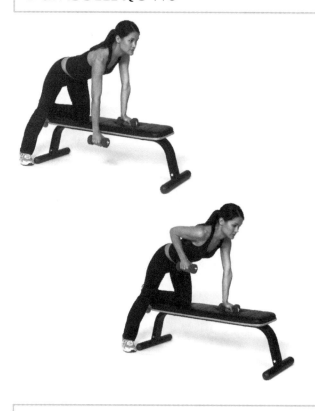

SETUP: Hold a dumbbell in each hand and place the same-side knee and hand on a stable bench. Keep your back flat throughout the movement.

MOVEMENT: Pull the weight up to just below your shoulder, concentrating on feeling a contraction in your mid-back on your working side. Hold that contraction for a moment, then slowly lower the weight. Feel the stretch in your back as you near the starting position. Perform all reps for one side before switching sides.

TRICEPS EXTENSIONS

TARGET: TRICEPS

SETUP: Sit on a balance ball or a flat or upright bench. Take a dumbbell in both hands, extend your arms up to the ceiling and let the weight dip behind your head. Your body should form a straight line from your hips to your elbows, with about a 90-degree bend at the elbows.

MOVEMENT: Press the weight up until your arms are extended toward the ceiling. Without locking out your elbows, contract the muscles along the backs of your arms for a moment. Return to the starting position.

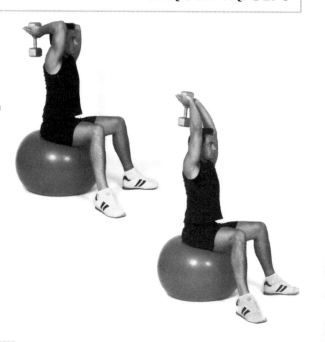

ALTERNATING CURLS

TARGET: BICEPS

SETUP: Stand, or sit on a balance ball or a flat bench, holding a dumbbell in each hand with your arms extended toward the ground and your palms facing each other.

MOVEMENT: Keeping your upper arm stationary, bring one weight up until your palm is facing your shoulder. Contract the muscles along the top of your arm for a moment. Lower the weight, feeling the stretch along the top of your arm. Switch to the other arm and perform a rep. Alternate arms until you have performed all the reps for each arm.

TUESDAY

Upper Body & Core

BALL CRUNCHES

TARGET: ABS

SETUP: Lie on a balance ball and plant your feet firmly on the floor. Lower your butt a couple of inches below your shoulders and knees. Place your hands behind your neck or lightly on the back of your head.

MOVEMENT: Use the strength of your mid-section to pull your upper body up until you feel a deep contraction in your midsection. Hold that for a moment. Return to the starting position.

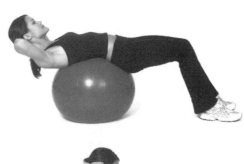

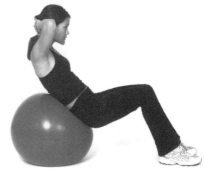

Tuesday option 2

Secondary Moves

Large muscle groups have primary and secondary movement functions. For instance, the primary movement of the pectorals is to press things away from the body. The secondary function of the pecs is to bring the arms across the body. This workout targets the secondary movement function of the major upper body muscles and the core. Training muscles for their secondary functions balances and strengthens the primary ones. It's a good idea to include this workout every third or fourth time you perform your Upper Body & Core Workout. These moves can be performed circuit-style, where you do one set of each move all the way through the list before performing a second set of any move, or you can perform all sets for one exercise before moving on to the next exercise.

EXERCISES	STARTER Sets/Reps	EXPERIENCED Sets/Reps
Chest Flyes	2/10	3/12
Lateral Raises	2/10	3/12
Reverse Back Extensions	2/10	3/12
Triceps Kickbacks	2/10	3/12
Hammer Curls	2/10	3/12
Cross-Body Twists	2/10	3/12

CHEST FLYES   TARGET: CHEST

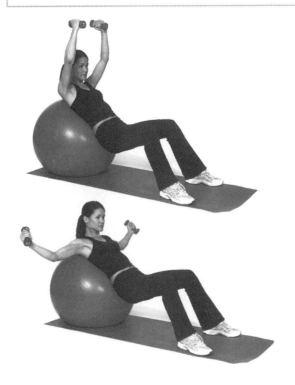

SETUP: Lie on a bench or balance ball with your feet firmly planted on the ground. Hold a dumbbell in each hand, palms facing one another. Extend the dumbbells directly above your shoulders. Maintain a slight bend at the elbows throughout the movement.

MOVEMENT: Lower the weights out to the side until the dumbbells are in the same plane as your torso (stop sooner if you feel pain or reach the limit of your range of motion). Feel the stretch across your chest. Bring the weights back up and contract your chest muscles. The dumbbells should be about 2 to 3 inches apart at the top of the movement.

LATERAL RAISES   TARGET: SHOULDERS

SETUP: Stand, or sit on a bench or balance ball, arms along your sides. Hold a dumbbell in each hand with your palms facing each other.

MOVEMENT: Raise the weights out to your sides until your arms are parallel to the ground. Contract your shoulder muscles for a moment. Fighting against gravity, slowly return to the starting position.

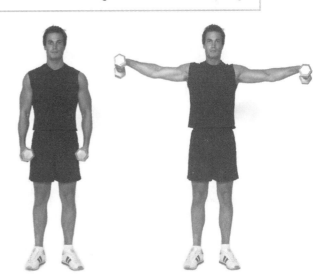

TUESDAY

Upper Body & Core

REVERSE BACK EXTENSIONS

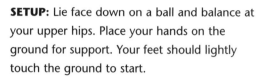

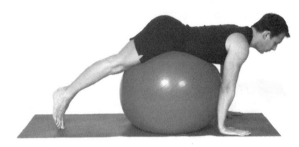

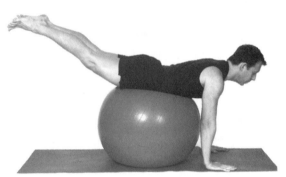

SETUP: Lie face down on a ball and balance at your upper hips. Place your hands on the ground for support. Your feet should lightly touch the ground to start.

MOVEMENT: Raise your feet until your lower body is parallel to the ground or a little higher; there should be no bend from your toes to hips. Slowly return to the starting position, allowing your toes to just touch the ground. Move directly into your next rep.

TRICEPS KICKBACKS

TARGET: TRICEPS

SETUP: Hold a dumbbell in each hand. Bend at the waist until your upper body roughly forms a 45-degree angle with the ground. Keep your spine in a neutral position—stick your butt out so there's no rounding of the lower back. With your arms by your sides, bend your elbows.

MOVEMENT: Moving only your lower arms, press the weights back until your arms form a straight line, from hand to shoulder. Contract the muscles at the backs of your arms. Slowly return to the starting position.

VARIATION: Perform this one arm at a time.

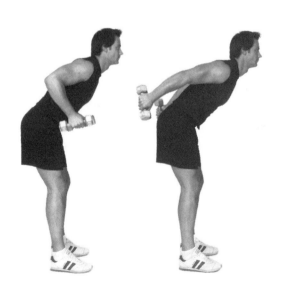

TUESDAY

Upper Body & Core

HAMMER CURLS   TARGET: BICEPS

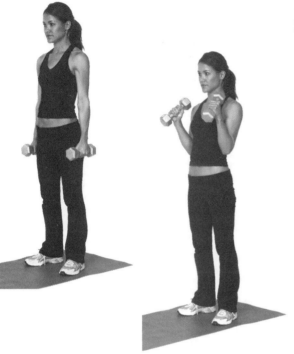

SETUP: Keeping your elbows by your sides, hold a dumbbell in each hand at waist level. Keep your palms facing one another at all times.

MOVEMENT: Raise both weights to your shoulders and contract the muscles on the sides of your arms for a moment. Return to the starting position, feeling the stretch along the outsides of your arms.

MODIFICATION: This can also be done while sitting.

CROSS-BODY TWISTS   TARGET: ABS

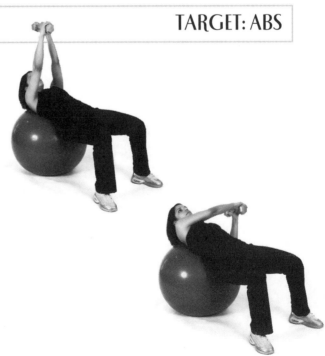

SETUP: Lie on your back on a balance ball and plant your feet firmly on the floor. Hold a weight in both hands directly overhead.

MOVEMENT: Slowly rotate your torso and move the weight out to one side, keeping your arms relatively straight. Maintain your spine in its neutral position and keep your neck extended with your gaze to the ceiling. Slowly return to the starting position and rotate to the other side, making certain to work within a range of motion that's comfortable for you.

Tuesday option 3

Major Muscle Groups

This workout adds a little more emphasis to the large muscles of the upper body—your chest, back and shoulders. It's a great option for those interested in adding a little more muscle mass. It's also a great way to include a little variety from one week to the next as it incorporates both primary and secondary moves. For this workout, perform all sets of one exercise before moving on to the next. This is a better muscle-building strategy than a circuit training–style workout. Also, for better muscle building and tone, use slightly heavier weights.

EXERCISES	STARTER Sets/Reps	EXPERIENCED Sets/Reps
Incline Chest Presses	2/10	3/12
Overhead Shoulder Presses	2/10	3/12
Dumbbell Rows	2/10	3/12
Chest Flyes	2/10	3/12
Front Raises	2/10	3/12
Floor Knee-Ups	2/10	3/12

INCLINE CHEST PRESSES

TARGET: CHEST

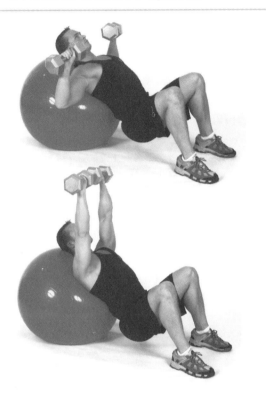

SETUP: This move can be performed on a balance ball or on an adjustable weight bench. Position yourself so that your upper body is at about a 45-degree angle, with your hips lower than your chest. Hold a dumbbell in each hand at your shoulder joint, elbows flared out.

MOVEMENT: Use the power of your chest to press the weights up toward the ceiling and contract the muscles of your chest as your arms reach full extension. Slowly lower the weights back to the starting position, feeling the stretch across your chest.

OVERHEAD SHOULDER PRESSES

TARGET: SHOULDERS

SETUP: Sit on a balance ball or a weight bench (the bench can be flat, or upright for more back support). Hold a dumbbell in each hand with your elbows near your sides and your hands just above shoulder height.

MOVEMENT: Press the weights up until your arms are fully extended. Without locking out your shoulders or elbows, contract the muscles on the sides of your shoulders for a moment. Return to the starting position, concentrating on feeling a stretch in your shoulders.

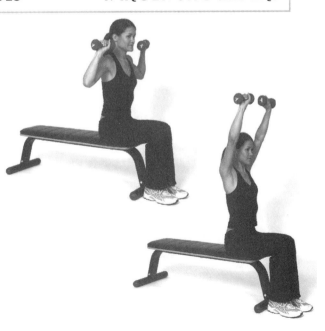

TUESDAY

Upper Body & Core

DUMBBELL ROWS 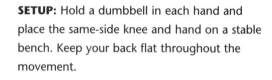 TARGET: BACK

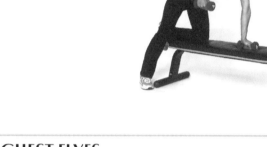

SETUP: Hold a dumbbell in each hand and place the same-side knee and hand on a stable bench. Keep your back flat throughout the movement.

MOVEMENT: Pull the weight up to just below your shoulder, concentrating on feeling a contraction in your mid-back on your working side. Hold that contraction for a moment, then slowly lower the weight. Feel the stretch in your back as you near the starting position. Perform all reps for one side before switching sides.

CHEST FLYES TARGET: CHEST

SETUP: Lie on a bench or balance ball with your feet firmly planted on the ground. Hold a dumbbell in each hand, palms facing one another. Extend the dumbbells directly above your shoulders. Maintain a slight bend at the elbows throughout the movement.

MOVEMENT: Lower the weights out to the side until the dumbbells are in the same plane as your torso (stop sooner if you feel pain or reach the limit of your range of motion). Feel the stretch across your chest. Bring the weights back up and contract your chest muscles. The dumbbells should be about 2 to 3 inches apart at the top of the movement.

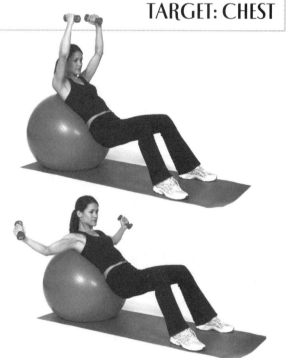

FRONT RAISES

TARGET: SHOULDERS

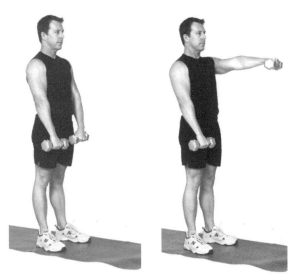

SETUP: Stand with your arms along the front of your body, holding a dumbbell in each hand with your palms facing your thighs.

MOVEMENT: Slowly raise one of the weights until your arm is parallel to the ground. Squeeze your shoulder muscles for a moment. Slowly return to the starting position then perform the same for the other side. Alternate arms until you have performed all reps for each arm.

FLOOR KNEE-UPS

TARGET: ABS

SETUP: Lie on the floor with your arms at your sides or lightly touching the back of your neck or head. Raise your straight legs and arms about an inch or two off the ground.

MOVEMENT: Bring your knees in toward your chest while you curl your upper body toward your knees. Crunch down on your midsection, then slowly extend your legs out until they are straight and hovering above the ground. Maintain the crunch for a second, then go directly into the next rep. Perform all reps before allowing your feet to contact the ground.

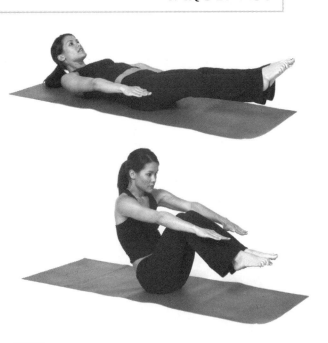

Tuesday option 4

Body Weight Moves

This workout uses your body weight instead of dumbbells, allowing you to strengthen your upper body by using your own weight. Many of these moves are even more challenging than their with-weight counterparts. While Starters can enjoy trying these moves, this option is better for more experienced exercisers. These moves can be performed circuit-style, where you do one set of each move all the way through the list before performing a second set of any move, or you can perform all sets for one exercise before moving on to the next exercise.

EXERCISES	STARTER Sets/Reps	EXPERIENCED Sets/Reps
Push-Ups	2/10	3/12
Bench Dips	2/10	3/12
Pull-Ups (Modified)	2/10	3/12
Pike Shoulder Presses	2/10	3/12
Roll-Up Crunches	2/10	3/12
Side Crunches	2/10	3/12

PUSH-UPS

TARGET: TRICEPS, CHEST

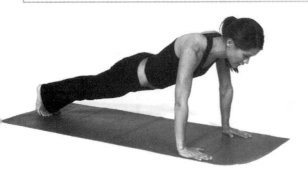

SETUP: Lie face down on the floor. Place your hands beneath your shoulders and push your body up until only your arms and feet are in contact with the ground. Your arms should be straight, and the rest of your body should form a diagonal line from your feet to the top of your head.

MOVEMENT: Bend at the elbows and shoulders to lower your body until your chest, chin or nose nearly touches the ground. Feel the stretch across your chest. Press back up to the staring position and contract your chest muscles. Perform reps slowly for more muscular stimulation while reducing the potential for injury.

MODIFICATION: To make the move easier, perform push-up sets from your knees and hands.

BENCH DIPS

TARGET: TRICEPS

SETUP: Sit on a weight bench and grab the edge of the bench closest to another piece of furniture, such as a chair. Place your feet on the chair. Move your butt up and away from the bench so that only your hands and lower limbs are supported.

MOVEMENT: Lower your butt below the padding of the bench, traveling down no further than the point where your upper arms are parallel to the ground. Feel the stretch along the backsides of your arms, then press up until your arms are straight, feeling the contraction along the backsides of your arms.

MODIFICATION: To make the move easier, start with your feet on the ground.

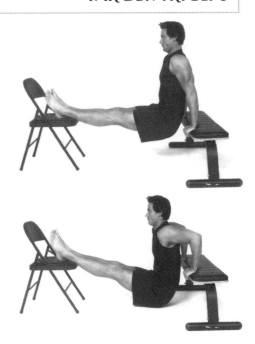

TUESDAY

Upper Body & Core

PULL-UPS

TARGET: CHEST, ARMS

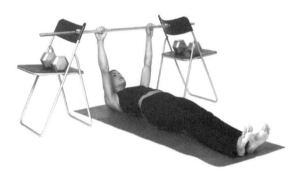

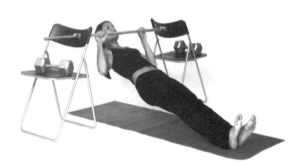

If you can perform standard pull-ups, include them in your workout. Many people cannot do the regular form but this is an excellent (but still challenging) version.

SETUP: Mount a stable bar about three to four feet off the ground. Hold onto the bar so that your body, from toes to head, lies in one plane and you're looking up at the ceiling. Your upper body should be able to hang with straight arms.

MOVEMENT: Pull your body up until your chest touches or comes close to the bar. Contract your back muscles, then lower back to the starting position.

MODIFICATION: To make the move easier, place the backs of your thighs on a bench or ball so you don't have to lift as much of your body weight for each rep.

PIKE SHOULDER PRESSES

TARGET: ARMS

SETUP: Place your hands on the ground about shoulder-width apart and your feet on a weight bench. Walk your upper body close to the bench so that your hips are as close to directly above your shoulders as is comfortable for you.

MOVEMENT: Bend your elbows and shoulders to lower yourself slowly before your head touches the ground, with your upper body perpendicular to the ground. Press back up until your arms are straight.

MODIFICATION: To make the move easier, place your shins or thighs on the bench.

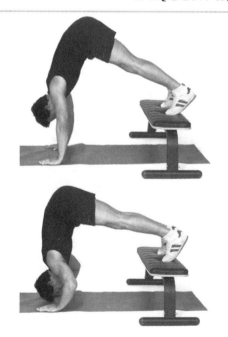

TUESDAY

Upper Body & Core

ROLL-UP CRUNCHES   TARGET: ABS

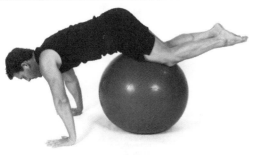

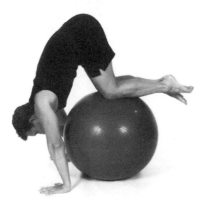

SETUP: Lie face down on the ball. Place the tops of your upper thighs on the ball and support your body weight with your hands out in front of you on the ground. Hold your arms straight and slightly wider than shoulder-width apart throughout the movement.

MOVEMENT: Without moving your hands, roll your knees toward your arms, allowing the ball to travel under you so that at the peak position it is under your lower legs at your knees. As you bring your knees in, your lower back and butt should curl upward. At the top of the movement, contract your abs for a moment. Slowly begin to roll the ball back, extending your legs behind you until you return to the starting position.

SIDE CRUNCHES   TARGET: ABS

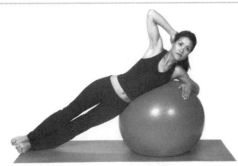

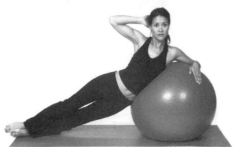

SETUP: Lie on your side on a balance ball or on the floor. For the ball version, stabilize yourself by pressing the edges of your feet into the ground. Place your lower arm on the ball, and the hand of the upper arm at the back of your head.

MOVEMENT: Pulling from your core, curl your upper body up and contract the muscles on the upper side of your body. Hold that contraction, then return to the starting position. Perform all the reps for one side, then switch sides.

Tuesday option 5

Easy Does It

Easy-Does-It workouts are for both Starter or Experienced exercisers—they can be used to help you grow more accustomed to regular exercise or to give you a break on days when you feel you need a less demanding workout. When you perform Easy-Does-It workouts, you can make modifications that suit your individual needs. You can reduce the amount of weight you use, eliminate a particular exercise, or perform fewer sets or reps. The purpose can be to get your heart rate up and make you feel a little livelier on a day when you are otherwise a bit sluggish.

EXERCISES	STARTER Sets/Reps	EXPERIENCED Sets/Reps
Chest Presses	2/10	3/12
Overhead Shoulder Presses	2/10	3/12
Preacher Curls	2/10	3/12
Lying Triceps Extensions	2/10	3/12
Side Crunches	2/10	3/12

CHEST PRESSES   TARGET: CHEST

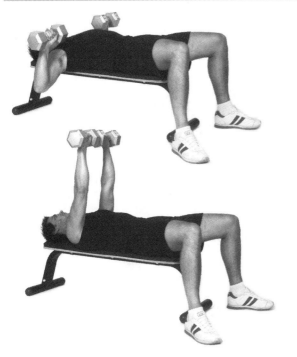

SETUP: Place the center of your back on a balance ball or lie on a flat weight bench. Hold a dumbbell in each hand near your armpits.

MOVEMENT: Use the strength of your chest to press the weights up until your arms are fully extended. Stop short of locking out your elbows and contract your chest muscles for a moment. Return to the starting position, concentrating on feeling a stretch across your chest.

OVERHEAD SHOULDER PRESSES   TARGET: SHOULDERS

SETUP: Sit on a balance ball or a weight bench (the bench can be flat, or upright for more back support). Hold a dumbbell in each hand with your elbows near your sides and your hands just above shoulder height.

MOVEMENT: Press the weights up until your arms are fully extended. Without locking out your shoulders or elbows, contract the muscles on the sides of your shoulders for a moment. Return to the starting position, concentrating on feeling a stretch in your shoulders.

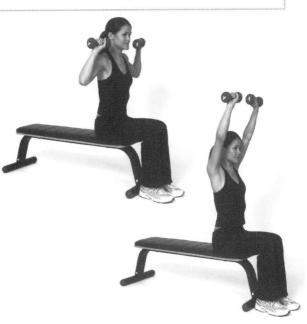

TUESDAY

Upper Body & Core

PREACHER CURLS   TARGET: BICEPS

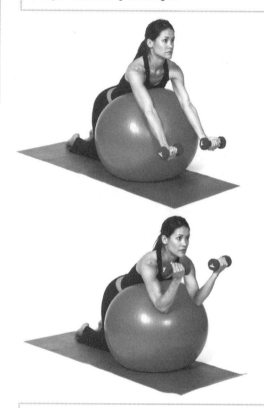

SETUP: Kneel in front of a balance ball with a dumbbell in each hand. Place the backs of each arm on the far side of the ball, with your arms outstretched and your palms facing up. Rotate your shoulders back as much as you can.

MOVEMENT: Moving only your lower arms and using the power of your biceps, pull the weights up toward your shoulders. At the top of the movement, contract your biceps for a moment. Lower the weights, feeling the stretch across the tops of your arms. Stop just short of fully extending your arms and begin the next rep.

LYING TRICEPS EXTENSIONS   TARGET: TRICEPS

SETUP: Lie on a bench, a balance ball or the ground. Hold a dumbbell in one hand and raise that arm until it is directly over your shoulder. Keep your upper arm stationary throughout the movement.

MOVEMENT: Bend your elbow and bring the weight toward your opposite shoulder. Stop before the weight touches your body, feeling a stretch across the backside of your working arm. Return to the starting position, contracting the muscles at the back of your arm as you reach the top. Perform all reps for this side of the body, then switch to the other side.

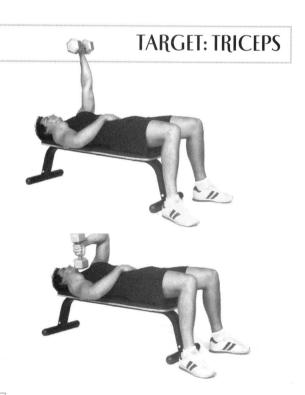

SIDE CRUNCHES

TARGET: ABS

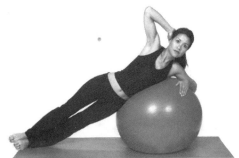

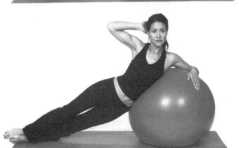

SETUP: Lie on your side on a balance ball or on the floor. For the ball version, stabilize yourself by pressing the edges of your feet into the ground. Place your lower arm on the ball, and the hand of the upper arm at the back of your head.

MOVEMENT: Pulling from your core, curl your upper body up and contract the muscles on the upper side of your body. Hold that contraction, then return to the starting position. Perform all the reps for one side, then switch sides.

Wednesday

flexibility workouts

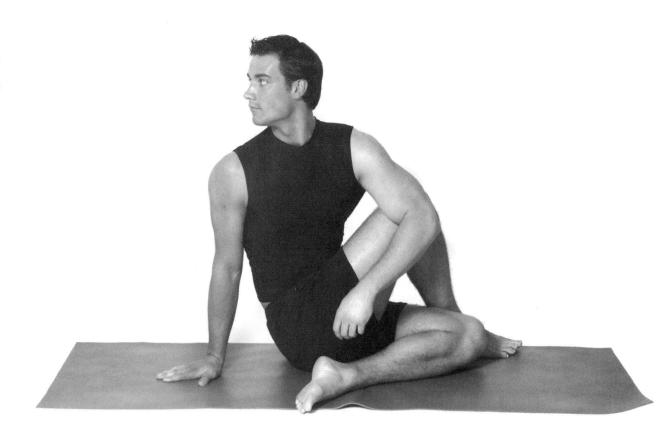

The Wednesday workouts give you three options. These include a standard stretching routine, a power movement flexibility workout and an easy-does-it flexibility workout. Feel free to include movements and variations for any of these flexibility workouts.

Also, feel free to add a few of your favorite flexibility moves to other training days, especially as a warm-up or cool-down. Finally, you can incorporate a second day of flexibility training each week, if desired, by doing it as your target-training (Saturday) workout.

OPTION 1	Standard Flexibility
OPTION 2	Power Movement Flexibility
OPTION 3	Easy-Does-It Flexibility

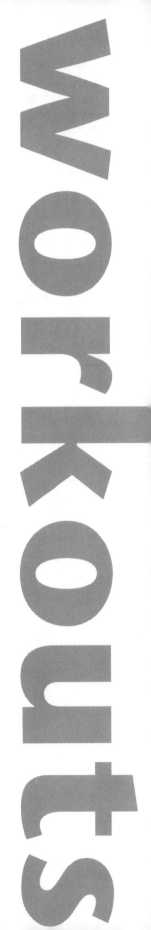

Wednesday option 1

Standard Flexibility

This workout incorporates many standard stretches. They should be performed in a slow fashion, holding each move for a few seconds or longer, depending on your skill level and the challenge of individual stretches. If you want to take your body through a wider range of motion, try the movement options as well.

Perform all reps for one set before moving on to the next move. After completing one set of all moves, Experienced trainers should return to the first move in the workout that is performed more than once (in this case, Forward Fold) and continue down the list until you have completed the requisite number of sets and reps for all stretches.

EXERCISES	STARTER Sets/Reps	EXPERIENCED Sets/Reps
Neck Rotation	1/4	1/4
Shoulder Rotation	1/4	1/4
Forward Fold	1/3	2/3
Warrior Stance	1/2	2/3
Side Lunge Stretch	1/2	2/3
Side Stretch	1/2	2/3
Down Dog	1/1	2/1
Lunge Stretch	1/2	2/3
Spinal Twist—Face Up	1/2	2/3
Shoulder Stretch/Child's Pose	1/1	2/1

NECK ROTATION

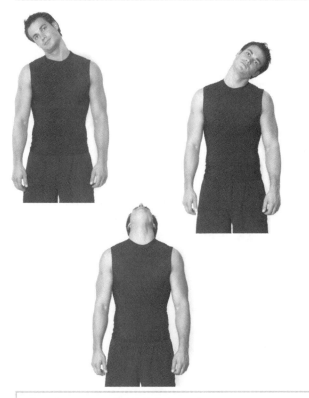

Primary benefits: stretches the neck and trapezius

MOVEMENT: Stand with your feet about hip-width apart and slowly roll your neck to one side. Allow your head to drop down toward your chest and roll your head to the other side. Finally drop your head back, opening your neck. Work slowly through this circle, making certain that you don't cause yourself discomfort or injury. After you have performed all your reps in one direction, perform neck rotations in the opposite direction.

SHOULDER ROTATION

Primary benefits: opens the shoulders

MOVEMENT: From standing, kneeling or sitting, extend one arm in front of you. Continue raising your arm until it's overhead. Allow it to stretch out and back. As soon as you complete a full circle with one side, complete a full rotation with the other. Alternate until you have completed all rotations for both sides, then reverse direction. Throughout, keep your movement slow and gentle.

VARIATION: Perform both arms at the same time.

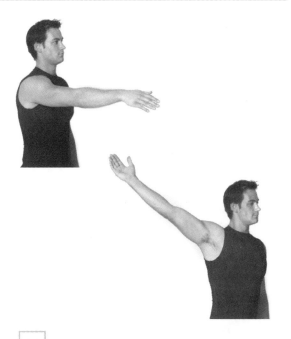

WEDNESDAY

Flexibility

FORWARD FOLD

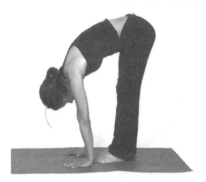

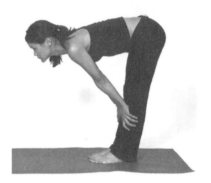

Primary benefits: stretches the glutes and hamstrings, elongates the spine

STRETCH: Stand with your feet together, or slightly wider if your hamstrings are tight. Keeping a slight arch in your lower back, bend from the waist; you can round your lower back as your head travels down until it is near or below your knees. Depending on your flexibility level, touch the ground, hold the backs of your legs or hold the opposite elbow in each hand. Hold your quads tight and allow the backs of your legs to open. Allow gravity to pull on your upper body, stretching your glutes and hamstrings. Slowly roll up your spine to the standing position.

MOVEMENT: While in the forward fold, press your hands against your shins or quads and raise your upper body until your back is flat.

WARRIOR STANCE

Primary benefits: multiple muscle stretch, strengthens the lower body

STRETCH: Stand with your feet together. Step forward with one foot until your knee is directly above your ankle. Turn your back foot so that it faces about 90 degrees out. Raise both arms straight up, palms facing one another. Hold as long as desired, then repeat on the other side.

MOVEMENT: Keeping your feet in place, rotate your upper body 90 degrees so that you are facing the side of the room. Lower your arms to shoulder height (this is the Warrior Two stance in yoga). Hold as long as desired, then return to the first stance. Repeat the sequence for the other side of the body.

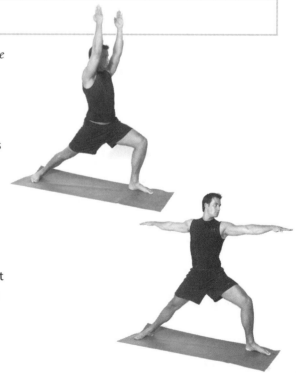

SIDE LUNGE STRETCH

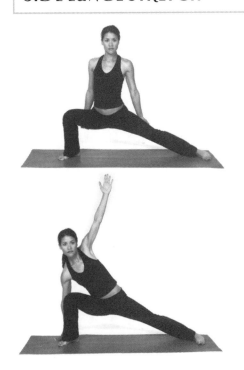

Primary benefits: stretches the inner thighs and lower legs

STRETCH: Stand with your feet wide apart. Keeping one leg straight, bend the other, allowing your hips to lower toward the foot on your bent-leg side. Maintain the natural curve in your back throughout the movement. Try to keep your upper body as upright as possible. Hold as long as desired. Repeat to the other side.

MOVEMENT: Stretch your arm on the straight-leg side up overhead as you bend your bent-knee side. The arm on your bent-leg side can touch the ground for support and to deepen the stretch. Allow your overhead arm to return to the starting position as you press back up to standing.

SIDE STRETCH

Primary benefits: excellent lateral whole-body stretch, working the legs, spine and shoulders

STRETCH: Stand with your legs about two to three feet apart. Keeping your body in one plane, bend at the waist to the left, allowing your left arm to drop toward your left leg as you stretch your right arm up and over your head. Think about elongating your spine as a way to allow for a deeper stretch. Hold as long as desired. Repeat on the opposite side.

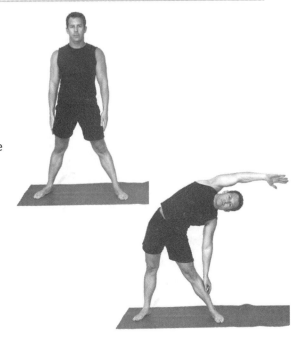

OPTION 1 — Standard Flexibility

DOWN DOG

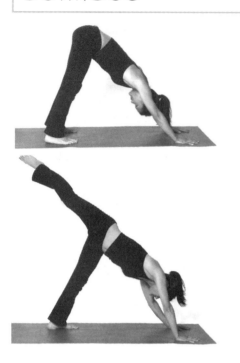

Primary benefits: stretches the whole body, particularly hamstrings and shoulders

STRETCH: Stand with your feet hip-width apart. Bend forward to place your hands on the ground then walk them forward, keeping your butt in the air. You should be straight from your heels to your hips and from your hands to your head to your hips; your heels can come off the ground. Essentially, you are in an inverted V position. In this position, work to keep the natural curvature in your lower back, full extension in your shoulder blades and your legs as straight as you can.

MOVEMENT: From Down Dog, slowly extend one leg up and behind you until your body forms a straight line from your hands through your raised leg. Lower and repeat on the other side.

LUNGE STRETCH

Primary benefits: stretches the hamstrings and quads

STRETCH: Stand with your feet together. Take a large step forward with one leg and bend your front knee, but don't let it travel out beyond your front foot. Allow your hips to sink until you feel a good stretch along the top of your trailing leg. (You can widen your feet as you get comfortable with the stance, placing your hands or knee on the ground to assist you if need be). Repeat on the opposite side.

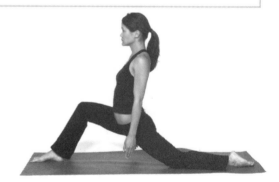

MOVEMENT: Twist to one side, placing your opposite elbow against the outside of your front leg, and press your hands together. (This twist works the spine and shoulders.)

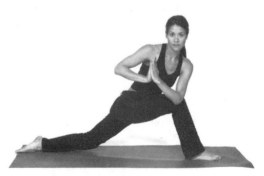

SPINAL TWIST—FACE UP

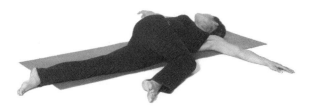

Primary benefits: elongates the spine, stretches the whole body

STRETCH: Lie on your back with your legs extended on the ground. Stretch your arms out to the sides and allow one knee to cross your body and drop to the side. Turn your head in the opposite direction of the knees and look out over your extended arm. Hold as long as desired, then return to center before repeating to the other side.

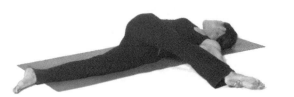

VARIATION: From the stretch position, slowly straighten your legs to deepen the stretch and to stretch your hamstrings as well. You may bring your top leg up and take a hold of it with the opposite arm to get a deeper stretch.

SHOULDER STRETCH/CHILD'S POSE

Primary benefits: relaxes the body, opens the shoulders

STRETCH: Lie face down with your hands beneath your shoulders. Push your hips back until your hamstrings are resting on your calves. Allow your weight to comfortably rest and sink into the ground. Keep your arms stretched overhead and, as your upper body sinks to the ground, feel a relaxing stretch in your shoulders. You can also rest your forehead on the ground. Hold as long as desired.

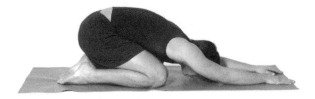

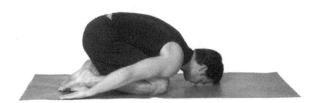

VARIATION: Place your arms along your sides or gently touch your feet.

Wednesday option 2

Power Movement Flexibility

This workout is more challenging—both in terms of its strength and flexibility demands—than the other flexibility workouts in this chapter. It includes many of the most challenging power moves such as the down dog power series and deeper stretches such as bridge and seated straddle stretch. You can also work to increase the difficulty of the workout by including many of the variations and movement options that make the basic moves more challenging.

Perform all reps for one set before moving on to the next move. After completing one set of all moves, Experienced trainers should return to the first move that has more than one set (in this case, Scoop Stretch to Arch) and continue down the list until you have completed the requisite number of sets and reps for all stretches. To make the work even more challenging, Experienced trainers can also add a third set of each of these repeated moves.

EXERCISES	STARTER Sets/Reps	EXPERIENCED Sets/Reps
Neck Rotation	1/4	1/4
Shoulder Rotation	1/4	1/4
Scoop Stretch to Arch	1/2	2/4
Down Dog Power Series	1/2	2/5
Straddle Stretch	1/2	2/3
Seated Press to Back Arch	1/2	2/4
Pigeon	1/2	2/2
Table Stretch	1/2	2/3
Bridge/Backbend	1/2	2/3
Shoulder Stretch/Child's Pose	1/1	2/1

NECK ROTATION

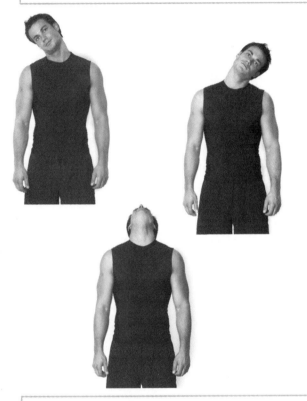

Primary benefits: stretches the neck and trapezius

MOVEMENT: Stand with your feet about hip-width apart and slowly roll your neck to one side. Allow your head to drop down toward your chest and roll your head to the other side. Finally drop your head back, opening your neck. Work slowly through this circle, making certain that you don't cause yourself discomfort or injury. After you have performed all your reps in one direction, perform neck rotations in the opposite direction.

SHOULDER ROTATION

Primary benefits: opens the shoulders

MOVEMENT: From standing, kneeling or sitting, extend one arm in front of you. Continue raising your arm until it's overhead. Allow it to stretch out and back. As soon as you complete a full circle with one side, complete a full rotation with the other. Alternate until you have completed all rotations for both sides, then reverse direction. Throughout, keep your movement slow and gentle.

VARIATION: Perform both arms at the same time.

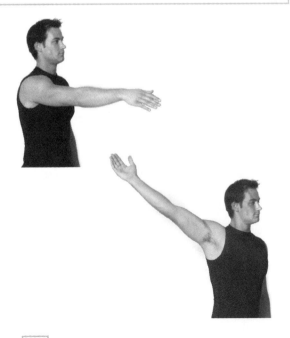

OPTION 2

Power Movement Flexibility

SCOOP STRETCH TO ARCH

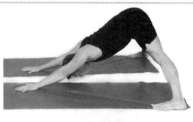
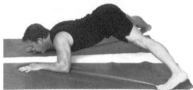
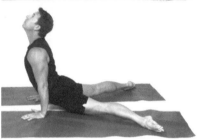

Primary benefits: stretches the whole body, strengthens upper body

SETUP: Stand with your legs as far apart as is comfortable for you. Bend at the waist and place your hands on the ground, walking them forward until your body is in one plane from your hips through your arms.

MOVEMENT: Drop your hips as you bend your arms and push your upper body forward, "scooping" through your arms. Begin to curve your lower back, allowing your upper body to rise with your legs spread wide (you can rest on the tops of your feet, or keep the bottoms in contact with the floor). Also, your thighs can rest against the ground, or you can hold them off the ground. Hold that position for as long as desired, then push back through each step until you are resting your weight back on your wide-spread legs in the starting position.

DOWN DOG POWER SERIES

Primary benefits: stretches and strengthens the whole body

SETUP: Begin in Down Dog (see page 94).

MOVEMENT: Slowly lower your hips until your body is in one plane from your feet to the top of your head. Lower down push-up style with your elbows by your sides, hovering just an inch or two off the ground for a moment (you can rest on your knees or the tops of your thighs). Press your chest forward and through your arms until your back is arched, resting only on your hands and the tops of your feet or the tops of your thighs. Press your hips back until you're in Down Dog. Hold the Down Dog for as long as desired before repeating the series.

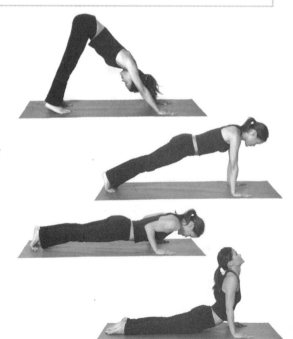

STRADDLE STRETCH

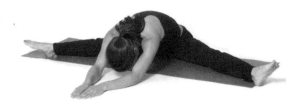

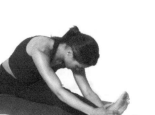

Primary benefits: stretches the upper legs, opens the hips, strengthens the lower back

STRETCH: Sit with your legs spread wide apart. Holding the natural curve in your back, fold forward and walk out your hands, supporting some of your upper body weight. Go as low as you can without straining or bending your legs. Hold as long as desired.

MOVEMENT: From the folded position, move your upper body toward your left leg and hold your foot, if possible. If you are quite flexible, stretch your right arm overhead until you can grasp your left foot with both hands. Repeat on the opposite side.

VARIATION: If you are very flexible, you can also move toward a full side-splits position and perform the above movement series.

SEATED PRESS TO BACK ARCH

Primary benefits: opens the shoulders, stretches the spine

SETUP: Sit with your legs spread wide apart. Reach one arm behind you and place it firmly on the ground

MOVEMENT: Press your hips up until your torso rises up off the ground and begins to arch. Stretch your other arm by your ear. Extend your body up as much as you can without creating discomfort or losing your balance. Then slowly lower your hips to the ground and repeat on the opposite side. Alternate until you have performed as many of these stretches as desired. Move slowly throughout this stretching movement to avoid overstretching or making yourself light-headed or dizzy.

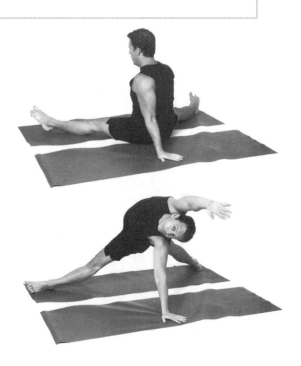

WEDNESDAY

Flexibility

PIGEON

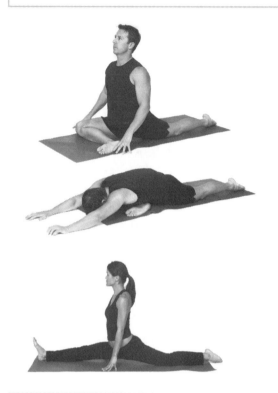

This is challenging, so start slowly to avoid injury. Primary benefits: opens the hips, stretches the quads and hamstrings

STRETCH: Kneel with your knees beneath your hips and your hands on the floor beneath your shoulders. Reach your right ankle toward your left wrist and stretch your left leg out behind you. Holding the normal arch in your lower back, sit upright, keeping your hips facing forward. Fold forward, walking your hands out to support your upper body. If you're flexible, you can allow your upper body to rest against your front leg while stretching your arms out overhead. Relax and sink into the stretch, holding it for as long as desired. Repeat on the other side.

VARIATION: If you're very flexible, straighten your front leg and work toward a full splits.

TABLE STRETCH

Primary benefits: opens the shoulders

STRETCH: Sit on the floor with your knees bent, feet flat on the floor, and your hands on the floor behind you. Gently press your body off the ground so that only your hands and feet contact the ground. Go up until your body is parallel to the ground. Hold as long as desired.

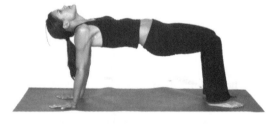

VARIATION: Remaining seated with your arms behind you, gently drop both knees to one side, feeling the stretch in the opposite shoulder. Bring your knees back to center, then repeat on the opposite side.

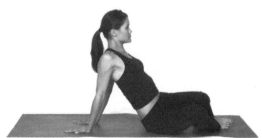

BRIDGE/BACKBEND

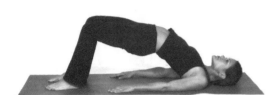

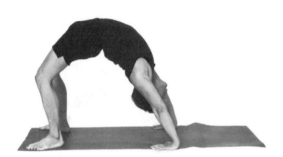

Primary benefits: opens the spine, stretches the lower back

STRETCH: Lie on your back with your arms at your sides and feet flat on the floor. Press through your feet to raise your butt off the ground. Tighten your buttocks to protect your lower back. Allow your shoulders to roll open to remove pressure from the back of your neck (rest your upper body weight on your shoulders rather than on the center of your back). Place your hands on the ground or at the base of your spine. Hold for as long as desired, then gently lower your hips back to the ground.

VARIATION: If you have enough flexibility and range of motion, place your hands on the ground by your ears and gently press up into a backbend. Tighten your butt to protect your lower back. Keep your feet parallel and your knees directly above your ankles.

SHOULDER STRETCH/CHILD'S POSE

Primary benefits: relaxes the body, opens the shoulders

STRETCH: Lie face down with your hands beneath your shoulders. Push your hips back until your hamstrings are resting on your calves. Allow your weight to comfortably rest and sink into the ground. Keep your arms stretched overhead and, as your upper body sinks to the ground, feel a relaxing stretch in your shoulders. You can also rest your forehead on the ground. Hold as long as desired.

VARIATION: Place your arms along your sides or gently touch your feet.

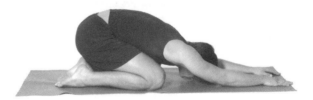

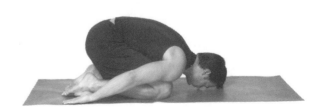

Wednesday option 3

Easy-Does-It Flexibility

This workout is designed as an easier—even soothing and relaxing—flexibility workout. It can also be performed as your mind/body workout on Sunday. While you can challenge yourself in many of these stretches, the purpose of this workout is to take it easy; make sure not to work at your full capacity—give your body a break. Then, when you want to work with a little more gusto, choose one of the more demanding flexibility workouts.

Perform all reps for one set before moving on to the next move. After completing one set of all moves, Experienced trainers should return to the first move that has more than one set (in this case, Cross-Leg Forward Fold) and continue down the list until you have completed the requisite number of sets and reps for all stretches.

EXERCISES	STARTER Sets/Reps	EXPERIENCED Sets/Reps
Neck Rotation (Seated)	1/4	1/4
Shoulder Rotation (Seated)	1/4	1/4
Cross-Leg Forward Fold	1/2	2/3
Seated Spinal Twist	1/2	2/3
Table Stretch (Seated)	1/2	2/3
Spinal Twist—Face Up	1/2	2/2
Spinal Twist—Face Down	1/2	2/2
Lying Hamstring Stretch	1/2	2/2
Forward Fold	1/2	2/2
Shoulder Stretch/Child's Pose	1/2	2/1

NECK ROTATION (SEATED)

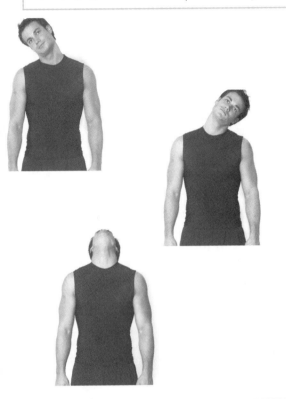

Primary benefits: stretches the neck and trapezius

MOVEMENT: Sit comfortably on a chair or on the floor and slowly roll your neck to one side. Allow your head to drop down toward your chest and roll your head to the other side. Finally drop your head back, opening your neck. Work slowly through this circle, making certain that you don't cause yourself discomfort or injury. After you have performed all your reps in one direction, perform neck rotations in the opposite direction.

SHOULDER ROTATION (SEATED)

Primary benefits: opens the shoulders

MOVEMENT: Sit or kneel comfortably and extend one arm in front of you. Continue raising your arm until it's overhead. Allow it to stretch out and back. As soon as you complete a full circle with one side, complete a full rotation with the other. Alternate until you have completed all rotations for both sides, then reverse direction. Throughout, keep your movement slow and gentle.

VARIATION: Perform both arms at the same time.

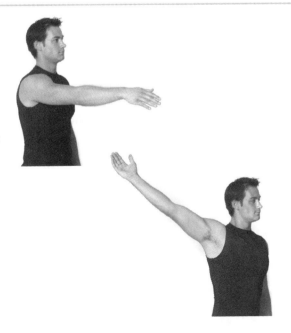

OPTION 3 — Easy-Does-It Flexibility

CROSS-LEG FORWARD FOLD

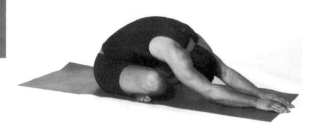

Primary benefits: strengthens the lower back, stretches the spine, opens the hips

STRETCH: Sit cross-legged on the ground. Bend as far forward as is comfortable, allowing your lower back to round and your hands to support your upper body as needed. As your upper body nears the ground, you can stretch your arms out overhead for a deeper stretch. Raise your upper body back up, supporting yourself with your hands against the ground as needed. Re-cross your legs with the opposite leg on the inside and perform the stretch again.

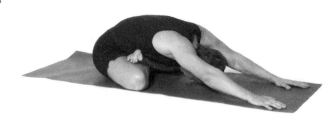

VARIATION: Perform this with your ankles resting on the opposite thigh or by pressing the soles of your feet together.

SEATED SPINAL TWIST

Primary benefits: strengthens the spine, opens the hips

STRETCH: Sit cross-legged on the ground. Keeping your posture as upright as possible, reach around and place one hand on the ground behind you. You can place your other hand against your opposite leg to support yourself and deepen the stretch, but be careful not to force your body into a too-deep stretch. Repeat to the other side.

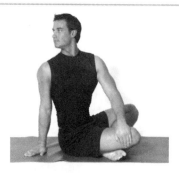

VARIATION: Raise the knee on the side that you're turning toward so that the bottom of your foot is on the ground. Place your same-side elbow against your knee as you reach behind you with the opposite hand.

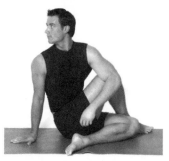

TABLE STRETCH (SEATED)

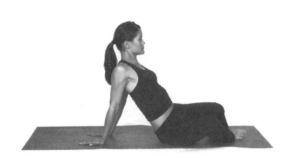

Primary benefits: opens the shoulders, stretches the hips

STRETCH: Sit on the floor with your knees bent, feet flat on the floor, and your hands on the floor behind you. Gently drop both knees to one side, feeling the stretch in the opposite shoulder. Bring your knees back to center, then repeat to the opposite side.

SPINAL TWIST—FACE UP

Primary benefits: elongates the spine, stretches the whole body

STRETCH: Lie on your back with your legs extended on the ground. Stretch your arms out to the sides and allow one knee to cross your body and drop to the side. Turn your head in the opposite direction of your knee and look out over your extended arm. Hold as long as desired, then return to center before repeating to the other side.

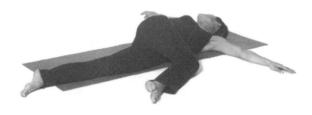

VARIATION: From the stretch position, slowly straighten your leg to deepen the stretch and to stretch your hamstrings as well. You may bring your top leg up and take a hold of it with the opposite arm to get a deeper stretch.

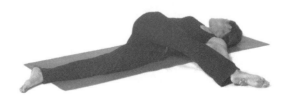

SPINAL TWIST—FACE DOWN

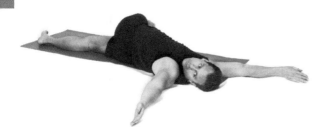

Primary benefits: stretches the spine and lower back

STRETCH: Lie face down with your arms extended above your head. Keeping the front side of your lower body in contact with the ground (you can spread your legs a couple of feet apart for more stability and leverage), allow your upper body to stretch open toward the ceiling. Return to the starting position and twist open to the other side. Keeping up a gentle moving pace is an excellent way to warm up the spine and lower back.

LYING HAMSTRING STRETCH

Primary benefits: stretches the hamstrings

STRETCH: Lie on your back with your legs extended along the floor. Raise one leg up and take hold of it with both hands. Hold your leg straight, feeling a stretch along your hamstrings. Keep your shoulders and head in contact with the ground. Hold as long as desired, then repeat on the other side

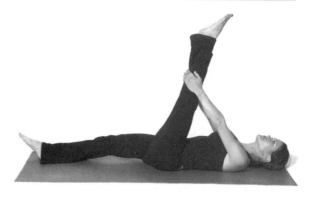

FORWARD FOLD

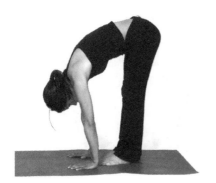

Primary benefits: stretches the glutes and hamstrings, elongates the spine

STRETCH: Stand with your feet together, or slightly wider if your hamstrings are tight. Keeping a slight arch in your lower back, bend from the waist; you can round your lower back as your head travels down until it is near or below your knees. Depending on your flexibility level, touch the ground, hold the backs of your legs or hold the opposite elbow in each hand. Hold your quads tight and allow the backs of your legs to open. Allow gravity to pull on your upper body, stretching your glutes and hamstrings. Slowly roll up your spine to the standing position.

SHOULDER STRETCH/CHILD'S POSE

Primary benefits: relaxes the body, opens the shoulders

STRETCH: Lie face down with your hands beneath your shoulders. Push your hips back until your hamstrings are resting on your calves. Allow your weight to comfortably rest and sink into the ground. Keep your arms stretched overhead and, as your upper body sinks to the ground, feel a relaxing stretch in your shoulders. You can also rest your forehead on the ground. Hold as long as desired.

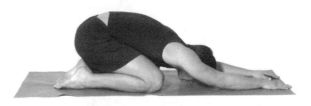

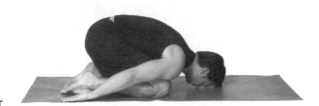

VARIATION: Place your arms along your sides or gently touch your feet.

Thursday

strength workouts— lower body & core

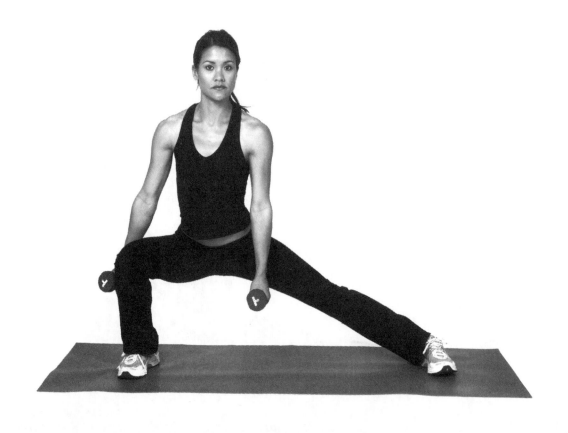

For your Thursday workouts, you are given five workout options. Each of these is an excellent lower body and core workout that you can complete in about 15 minutes. Choose the one that appeals to you most on any given Lower Body & Core training day. One week, you may feel like doing the standard moves Workout 1. Another day you may feel more like trying the power circuit Workout 4. Perform whichever workout you want from this chapter on your Thursday lower-body strength-training day. It's a great idea to change from one workout to another from one week to the next, but you'll also get great results if you find you like one workout better than the others, and simply want to do that workout on any given Thursday.

OPTION 1	Standard Moves
OPTION 2	Challenging Moves
OPTION 3	Unilateral Moves
OPTION 4	Lower-Body Power Circuit
OPTION 5	Easy-Does-It Moves

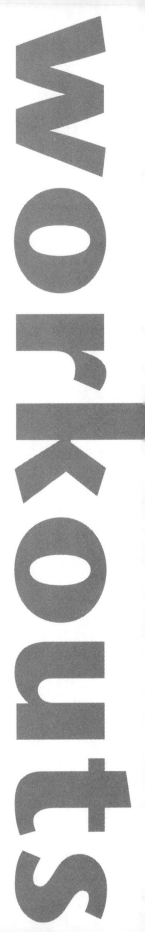

Thursday option 1

Standard Moves

This workout includes some of the most standard lower-body weight-training moves, making it a great primary workout for your lower body. This workout also includes two core moves, while other workouts only include one or none. As such, this is an excellent choice for targeting your abs as well as your butt and thighs. Do all sets of one movement before moving on to the next exercise. If you prefer the circuit type of training, then perform Option 4 instead.

EXERCISES	STARTER Sets/Reps	EXPERIENCED Sets/Reps
Squats	2/10	3/15
Stiff-Legged Deadlifts	2/10	3/15
Calf Raises	2/10	3/15
Floor Crunches	2/10	3/15
Floor Knee-Ups	2/10	3/15

SQUATS

TARGET: QUADS

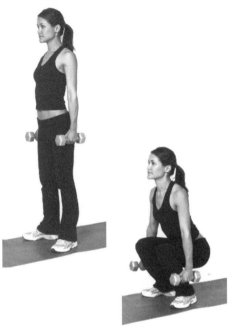

SETUP: Stand with your feet about hip-width apart. Your toes can angle outward a bit if that helps you deepen the move and allows you to feel more stable. Hold a dumbbell in each hand at your sides. Maintain the natural curve in your lower back throughout the move.

MOVEMENT: Bend at both the knees and hips, allowing the weights to drift toward the floor. Push your butt back as you drop down to keep your knees from traveling too far forward. Go down as low as is comfortable, feeling a stretch along the backs of your legs and a contraction across the top. Press evenly through your heels and toes to rise back up to the starting position.

STIFF-LEGGED DEADLIFTS

TARGET: HAMSTRINGS, BUTT

SETUP: Stand with your feet a little closer than hip-width apart, either with your legs straight or with a slight break at the knees, but hold that position throughout the move. Hold a dumbbell in each hand, or use a barbell or broomstick. Maintain the natural curve in your lower back throughout the move.

MOVEMENT: Bend forward from the waist; avoid bending at the knees. Allow the weights to travel out in front of your legs as you bend, lowering down until your upper body is parallel to the ground. Stop before your lower back begins to round. Feel the stretch across the backs of your legs and butt as you pause for a moment. Drive through your heels and toes to slowly return to the starting position. Contract the muscles at the backs of your legs at the top of the move.

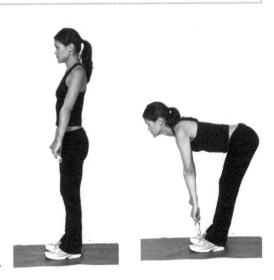

THURSDAY

Lower Body & Core

CALF RAISES

TARGET: CALVES

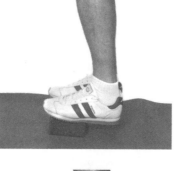

SETUP: Using a block near a wall or a stairway with a rail, stand on the edge of the block or step with the fronts of both feet, letting your heels hang over. Keep both legs straight throughout the movement.

MOVEMENT: Rise onto your toes and feel the contraction at the backs of your lower legs. Slowly lower both heels until they're below your toes, feeling a good stretch at the backs of your lower legs.

VARIATION: For added resistance, hold a weight.

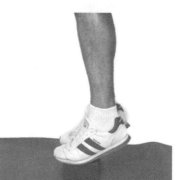

FLOOR CRUNCHES

TARGET: ABS

SETUP: Lie on the floor and place both feet flat on the floor, relatively close to your butt. Place your hands lightly at the back of your head or base of your neck.

MOVEMENT: Using the power of your midsection, raise your upper body a few inches off the ground, curling your head toward your knees. Feel the contraction in the center of your abs for a moment. Still holding that area taut, return to the starting position.

ADVANCED MODIFICATION: Place your feet against the wall with your lower legs parallel to the ground. Your upper legs should be close to perpendicular to the ground.

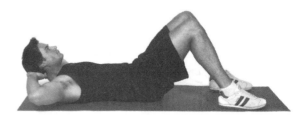

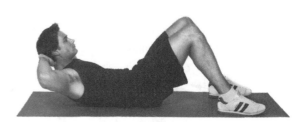

FLOOR KNEE-UPS

TARGET: ABS

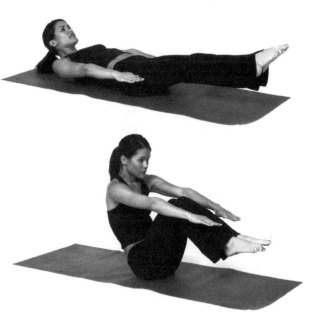

SETUP: Lie on the floor with your arms at your sides or lightly touching the back of your neck or head. Raise your straight legs and arms about an inch or two off the ground.

MOVEMENT: Bring your knees in toward your chest while you curl your upper body toward your knees (you can stop short of allowing them to touch, at the point where you feel the most effort in your abs). Crunch down on your midsection, then slowly extend your legs out until they are straight and hovering above the ground. Maintain the crunch for a second, then go directly into the next rep. Perform all reps before allowing your feet to contact the ground.

Thursday option 2

Challenging Moves

This workout consists of standard exercises for the lower body and core, but it is a more challenging workout than Option 1, relying on some of the more difficult exercises and variations. Do this workout on days when you feel motivated and energetic.

Perform all reps for one set before moving on to the next move. After completing one set of all moves, return to the top of the list and continue down the list until you have completed the requisite number of sets and reps for all exercises.

EXERCISES	STARTER Sets/Reps	EXPERIENCED Sets/Reps
Squats (Weights Overhead)	2/10	3/15
Alternating Lunges	2/10	3/15
Deadlifts	2/10	3/15
Calf Raises (One Leg)	2/10	3/15
V-Pike Raises	2/10	3/15

THURSDAY

Lower Body & Core

SQUATS (WEIGHTS OVERHEAD)　　TARGET: QUADS

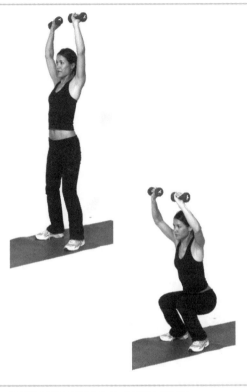

SETUP: Stand with your feet about hip-width apart. Hold a dumbbell in each hand and press them overhead until your arms are almost fully extended. Maintain this arm position as well as the natural curve in your lower back throughout the movement.

MOVEMENT: Bend at the hips and knees to squat down, holding your core tight to provide additional stability. Go as low as taking your upper legs parallel to the ground. Feel the stretch across the backs of your legs and butt, and the contraction along the fronts of your legs. Press evenly through your heels and toes to rise back up to the starting position.

MODIFICATIONS: Instead of holding the weights overhead, hold the weights at shoulder height. You can also modify the move by extending your arms overhead without weights.

ALTERNATING LUNGES　　TARGET: LEGS

SETUP: Stand with your feet together. Hold a dumb-bell in each hand. Keep your shoulders rotated back and your spine neutral throughout the move.

MOVEMENT: Take a large step forward and sink down, letting the weights travel toward the ground. The thigh of your front leg should come close to parallel, but you need not go as low as parallel. Pressing evenly through the toes and heel of your front foot, step your front leg back to the starting position. Repeat on the other side.

VARIATION: Perform walking lunges by stepping forward, dropping your hips, then pressing through your back foot. Step with the other foot and continue. You will need space for this move.

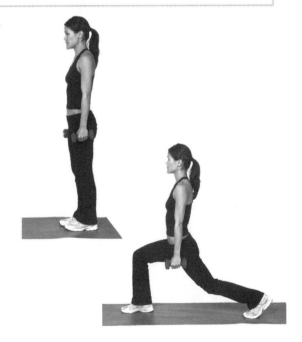

THURSDAY

Lower Body & Core

DEADLIFTS

TARGET: LEGS, BUTT

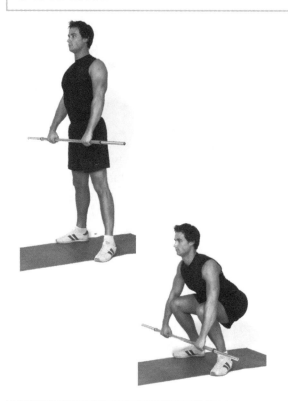

SETUP: Stand with your legs slightly wider than hip-width apart; your toes can point outward a bit if this gives you more stability. Hold a barbell or broomstick, with your hands slightly farther apart than body width. Keep your lower back neutral throughout the movement.

MOVEMENT: Squat down, allowing the barbell or broomstick to travel out beyond your knees. Go as low as you can (you may be able to take your butt almost all the way to the ground). Feel the stretch in your glutes and lower legs and the contraction along the tops of your legs. Press evenly through your heels and toes to return to the standing position. Contract the backs of your legs and glutes as you reach the top.

CALF RAISES (ONE LEG)

TARGET: CALVES

SETUP: Using a block near a wall, or a stairway with a rail, stand on the edge of the block or step with the front of one foot, letting that heel hang over. Hold your other foot off the ground behind you or curl it against the ankle of the working leg. Keep your working leg straight throughout the movement.

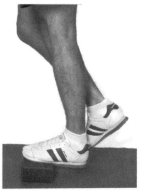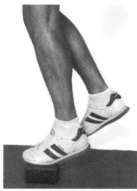

MOVEMENT: Rise onto your toes and feel the contraction at the back of your lower leg. Slowly lower your heel until its below your toes, feeling a good stretch at the back of your lower leg. Perform all reps for one leg, then switch sides.

VARIATION: For added resistance, hold a weight.

THURSDAY

V-PIKE RAISES   TARGET: ABS

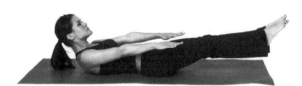

SETUP: Lie on your back and raise your legs a couple of inches off the ground. Holding the natural curve in your lower back as much as you can, also bring your upper body an inch or so off the ground.

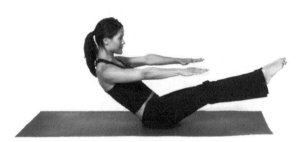

MOVEMENT: Simultaneously raise your straight legs and upper body while extending your arms toward your toes. With control, lower your body back down to the starting position. Avoid letting either your upper body or legs touch the ground—stay balanced on your butt throughout the move.

Lower Body & Core

Thursday option 3

Unilateral Moves

For this workout, you will work each leg separately from the other, either performing all moves for one side of the body and then for the other; or else alternating work for one side of the body with the other. Unilateral moves are excellent for enhancing balance and power. For example, performing lunges all on one side first, then the other, enables you to work each leg with more intensity since you don't let it rest between reps. However, since you may feel more fatigued on the second leg than you do for the first, alternate your starting leg from one workout to the next (if you start with your left leg this week, start with your right next week).

Perform all reps for one set before moving on to the next move. After completing one set of all moves, return to the top of the list and continue down the list until you have completed the requisite number of sets and reps for all exercises.

EXERCISES	STARTER Sets/Reps	EXPERIENCED Sets/Reps
Lunges	2/10	3/15
Alternating Back Lunges	2/10	3/15
Side Lunges	2/10	3/15
Calf Raises (One Leg)	2/10	3/15
Side Crunches	2/10	3/15

LUNGES

TARGET: LEGS

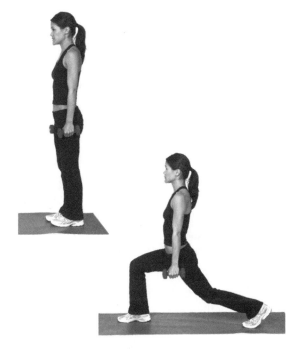

SETUP: Stand with your feet together and hold a dumbbell in each hand at your sides. Keep your shoulders rotated back and your spine neutral throughout the move.

MOVEMENT: Take a large step forward and sink down, letting the weights travel toward the ground. Your upper thigh should come close to parallel. Feel the stretch in the back of your front leg and across the front of your back leg. Press evenly through the toes and heel of your front foot to step back to the starting position. Complete all reps for one leg before doing the same for the other.

MODIFICATION: Stand with your legs in the lunging position and simply sink down and press up without including the stepping motion.

ALTERNATING BACK LUNGES

TARGET: LEGS

This excellent complement to forward lunging encourages all-around lower-body strength and development.

SETUP: Stand with your feet together and hold a dumbbell in each hand at your sides. Keep your shoulders rotated back and your spine neutral throughout the move.

MOVEMENT: Take a large step backward and sink down, letting the weights travel toward the ground. The thigh of your front leg should come close to parallel. Feel the stretch in the back of your front leg and across the front of your back leg. Push up and forward through your back foot, allowing you to return to the starting position. Alternate sides until you have completed all appointed reps.

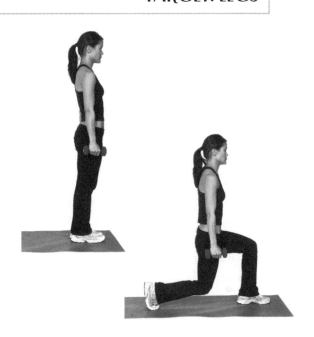

119

OPTION 3   Unilateral Moves

SIDE LUNGES   TARGET: LEGS

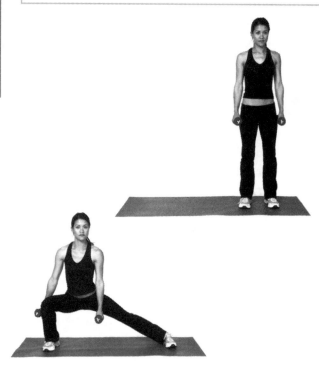

At first, you may want to perform these without holding weights since these require more balance than the other lunges.

SETUP: Stand with your feet together and your shoulders rolled back. Hold your spine neutral throughout the movement.

MOVEMENT: Step about three feet out to one side and drop your hips down toward your traveling leg. Your upper body can come forward as you lower your body toward the ground, but only go as low as is comfortable, and avoid ballistic or sudden moves. At the low point of the move, your foot should be flat on the ground. Press back up through the toes and heel of the traveling leg. Return to the starting position, then alternate sides until you have completed all reps for each side.

CALF RAISES (ONE LEG)   TARGET: CALVES

SETUP: Using a block near a wall, or a stairway with a rail, stand on the edge of the block or step with the front of one feet, letting that heel hang over. Hold your other foot off the ground behind you or curl it against the ankle of the working leg. Keep your working leg straight throughout the movement.

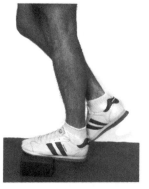
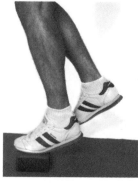

MOVEMENT: Rise onto your toes and feel the contraction at the back of your lower leg. Slowly lower your heel until its below your toes, feeling a good stretch at the back of your lower leg. Perform all reps for one leg, then switch and do the same for the other leg.

VARIATION: For added resistance, hold a weight.

SIDE CRUNCHES

TARGET: ABS

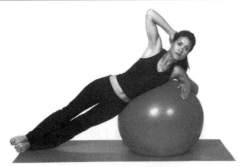

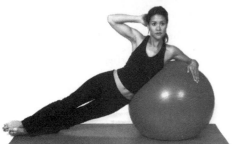

SETUP: Lie on your side on a balance ball or on the floor. For the ball version, stabilize yourself by pressing the edges of your feet into the ground. Place your lower arm on the ball, and the hand of the upper arm at the back of your head.

MOVEMENT: Pulling from your core, curl your upper body up and contract the muscles on the upper side of your body. Hold that contraction, then return to the starting position. Perform all the reps for one side, then switch sides.

Thursday option 4

Lower-Body Power Circuit

This workout is designed to be done circuit style, where you perform one set of each exercise, then cycle through the exercises again until you have completed the requisite number of sets for your program. Note that this workout does not contain a core move. Feel free to add one in after you have completed all sets for your legs power circuit (good choices are floor or ball crunches). At first, this should prove challenging, so rest as needed between sets. Work up to performing the entire workout without rest.

EXERCISES	STARTER Sets/Reps	EXPERIENCED Sets/Reps
Squats	2/10	3/15
Alternating Lunges	2/10	3/15
Squats (Weights Overhead)	2/10	3/15
Stiff-Legged Deadlifts	2/10	3/15
Calf Raises	2/10	3/15

Lower-Body Power Circuit

SQUATS   TARGET: QUADS

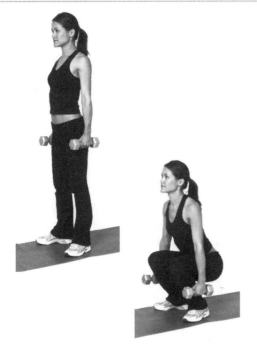

STARTING POSITION: Stand with your feet about hip-width apart. Your toes can angle outward a bit if that helps you deepen the move and allows you to feel more stable. Hold a dumbbell in each hand at your sides. Maintain the natural curve in your lower back throughout the move.

MOVEMENT: Bend at both the knees and hips, allowing the weights to drift toward the floor. Push your butt back as you drop down to keep your knees from traveling too far forward. Go down as low as is comfortable, feeling a stretch along the backs of your legs and a contraction across the top. Press evenly through your heels and toes to rise back up to the starting position.

ALTERNATING LUNGES   TARGET: LEGS

SETUP: Stand with your feet together. Hold a dumbbell in each hand. Keep your shoulders rotated back and your spine neutral throughout the move.

MOVEMENT: Take a large step forward and sink down, letting the weights travel toward the ground. The thigh of your front leg should come close to parallel, but you need not go as low as parallel. Pressing evenly through the toes and heel of your front foot, step your front leg back to the starting position. Repeat on the other side.

VARIATION: Perform walking lunges by stepping forward, dropping your hips, then pressing through your back foot. Step with the other foot and continue. You will need space for this move.

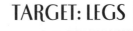
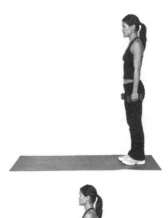
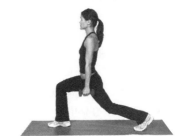

THURSDAY

Lower Body & Core

SQUATS (WEIGHTS OVERHEAD)   TARGET: QUADS

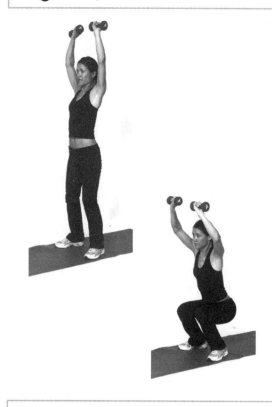

SETUP: Stand with your feet about hip-width apart. Hold a dumbbell in each hand and press them overhead until your arms are almost fully extended. Maintain this arm position as well as the natural curve in your lower back throughout the movement.

MOVEMENT: Bend at the hips and knees to squat down, holding your core tight to provide additional stability. Go as low as taking your upper legs parallel to the ground. Feel the stretch across the backs of your legs and butt, and the contraction along the fronts of your legs. Press evenly through your heels and toes to rise back up to the starting position.

STARTER MODIFICATIONS: Hold the weights at shoulder height instead of overhead. You can also modify the move by extending your arms overhead without weights.

STIFF-LEGGED DEADLIFTS   TARGET: HAMSTRINGS, BUTT

SETUP: Stand with your feet a little closer than hip-width apart, either with your legs straight or with a slight break at the knees, but hold that position throughout the move. Hold a dumbbell in each hand, or use a barbell or broomstick. Maintain the natural curve in your lower back throughout the move.

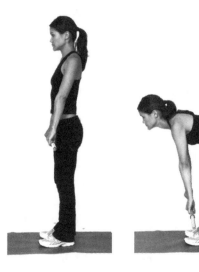

MOVEMENT: Bend forward from the waist; avoid bending at the knees. Allow the weights to travel out in front of your legs as you bend, lowering down until your upper body is parallel to the ground. Stop before your lower back begins to round. Feel the stretch across the backs of your legs and butt as you pause for a moment. Drive through your heels and toes to slowly return to the starting position. Contract the muscles at the backs of your legs at the top of the move.

CALF RAISES

TARGET: CALVES

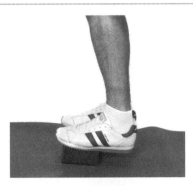

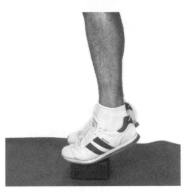

SETUP: Using a block near a wall or a stairway with a rail, stand on the edge of the block or step with the fronts of both feet, letting your heels hang over. Keep both legs straight throughout the movement.

MOVEMENT: Rise onto your toes and feel the contraction at the backs of your lower legs. Slowly lower both heels until they're below your toes, feeling a good stretch at the backs of your lower legs.

VARIATION: For added resistance, hold a weight.

Thursday option 5

Easy-Does-It Moves

This is a great workout for beginners or advanced strength trainers who want an easier day. Often, this is a great strategy when you're sore from other workouts or activities, feeling a little sluggish or trying to stay active while coping with a minor injury (if injured, however, always seek a doctor's advice before pursuing any type of exercise regimen). All the moves in this workout can be performed with or without weights.

EXERCISES	STARTER Sets/Reps	EXPERIENCED Sets/Reps
Squats (Partial)	2/10	3/15
Lunges (Partial)	2/10	3/15
Stiff-Legged Deadlifts (Partial)	2/10	3/15
Calf Raises (Partial)	2/10	3/15
Ball Crunches	2/10	3/15

SQUATS (PARTIAL)   TARGET: QUADS

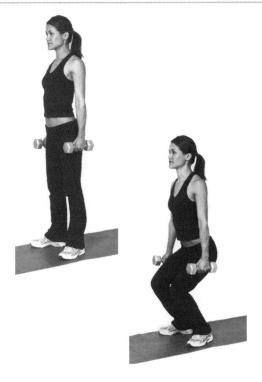

SETUP: Stand with your feet about hip-width apart, arms at your sides. Your toes can angle outward a bit if that helps you deepen the move and allows you to feel more stable. Hold a dumbbell in each hand at your sides. Maintain the natural curve in your lower back throughout the move.

MOVEMENT: Bend at both the knees and hips to lower to the floor. Push your butt back as you drop down to keep your knees from traveling too far forward. Go down only halfway to parallel, where your upper legs make about a 45-degree angle with the ground. Press evenly through your heels and toes to rise back up to the starting position.

MODIFICATION: Perform this without weights.

LUNGES (PARTIAL)   TARGET: LEGS

SETUP: Stand with one foot about three feet in front of the other. Keep this foot position throughout the movement. Hold a dumbbell in each hand at your sides.

MOVEMENT: Allow your hips to drop about six to eight inches, making sure that your hips stay higher than your knees. Press back up to the starting position. Perform all reps for one side of the body, then switch and perform all reps for the other side.

MODIFICATION: Perform this without weights.

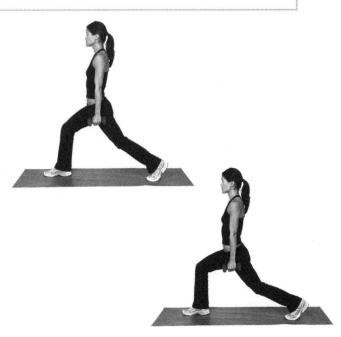

THURSDAY

Lower Body & Core

STIFF–LEGGED DEADLIFTS (partial)   TARGET: HAMSTRINGS, BUTT

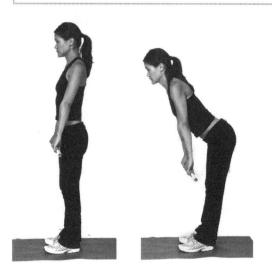

SETUP: Stand with your feet a little closer than hip-width apart and hold a dumbbell in each hand, or use a barbell or broomstick. Bend your knees slightly, maintaining this bend and the neutral curve of your lower back throughout the move.

MOVEMENT: Bend forward from the waist but avoid bending more at the knees. Allow the weights to travel out in front of your legs as you bend. Lower down until your upper body forms about a 45-degree angle with ground. Press through your heels and toes to slowly return to the standing position.

MODIFICATION: Perform this without weights.

CALF RAISES (PARTIAL)   TARGET: CALVES

SETUP: Using a block near a wall, or a stairway with a rail, stand on the edge of the block or step with the fronts of both feet, letting your heels hang over. Keep both legs straight throughout the move.

MOVEMENT: Rise onto your toes about an inch or so and feel the contraction at the backs of your lower legs. Slowly lower both heels until they are level with your toes.

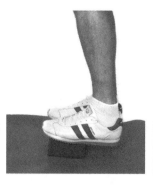
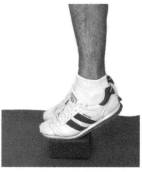

BALL CRUNCHES   TARGET: ABS

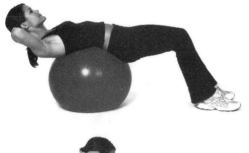

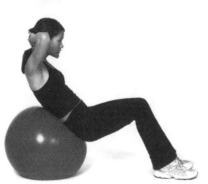

SETUP: Lie on a balance ball and plant your feet firmly on the floor. Lower your butt a couple of inches below your shoulders and knees. Place your hands behind your neck or lightly on the back of your head.

MOVEMENT: Use the strength of your midsection to pull your upper body up until you feel a deep contraction in your midsection. Hold that for a moment. Return to the starting position.

Friday

cardio workouts

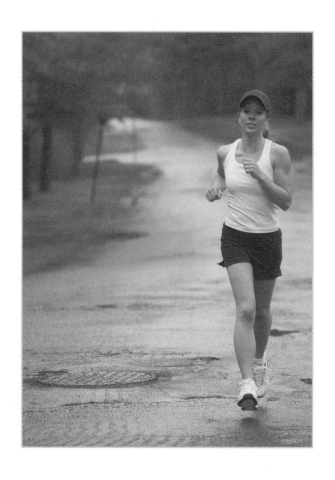

The Fit in 15 program offers eight different cardiovascular options to choose from for your Monday and Friday workouts. For detailed information on the types of training, turn to page 58.

Consider mixing up your workouts from one session to another. It's also a great idea to change the pace at which you work. Some days, you may have a lot of energy and might want to include a few minutes of light jogging with your brisk walk. On days when you're less energetic or you feel like you're still a little sore from the workouts of the previous days, you might consider an easy-does-it walk.

OPTION 1	Brisk Walking
OPTION 2	Light Jogging/Running
OPTION 3	Bicycling
OPTION 4	Swimming
OPTION 5	Water Walking/Aerobics
OPTION 6	Treadmill
OPTION 7	Other Exercise Equipment
OPTION 8	Easy-Does-It Walking

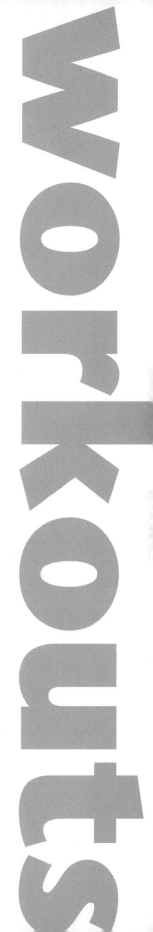

Saturday

target-training workouts

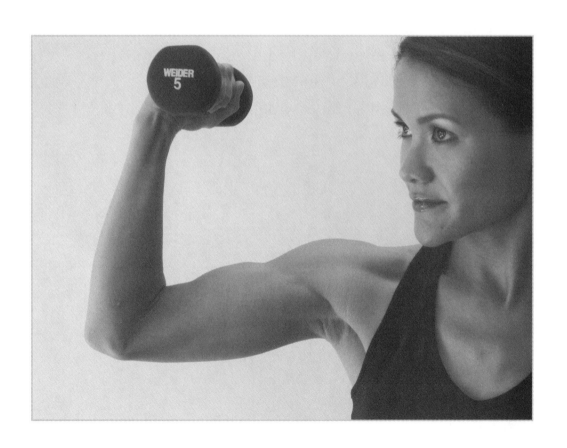

Target Training workouts on Saturday really allow you to individualize your Fit in 15 program. On this day, you can choose any workout from this chapter or any other in the book to emphasize any form of training to get the results you want most. For instance, you may want to emphasize firming your midsection or arms. This Target Training chapter provides a workout that directly targets each of these, allowing you to emphasize either of these body parts in your training.

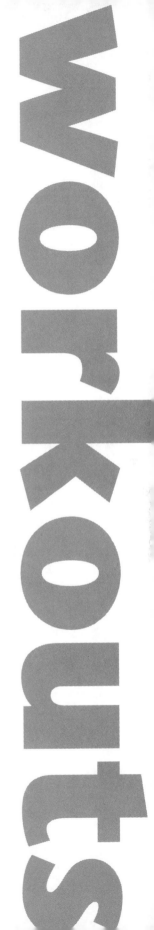

OPTION 1	Arm-Toning Workout
OPTION 2	Butt-Firming Workout
OPTION 3	Thigh-Tightening Workout
OPTION 4	Body Fat–Reducing Workout
OPTION 5	Upper-Body Workout
OPTION 6	Abs-Developing Workout
OPTION 7	Flexibility Workout
OPTION 8	Cardio Workout

1. ARM-TONING WORKOUT

If toned arms are your goal, then, in addition to your regular strength-training workouts, you should also perform this workout, which consists of arms exercises with weights. Each Saturday, perform these biceps and triceps moves. The workout begins with the triceps, the muscles at the back of the arm. The triceps are a larger muscle group than the biceps, which you will also work. Hammer curls emphasize the brachialis, which lies between the biceps and triceps. Including all these moves one additional time a week will help you more fully develop and tone your arms.

2. BUTT-FIRMING WORKOUT

If you're one of the many people who want a firmer back end, then use the Butt-firming Workout on your Target Training Saturdays. Perform all sets of one exercise before moving on to the next, or perform them circuit style, where you do one set of each exercise before returning to the first exercise for your second set. Continue working from the first exercise to the last until you have performed all sets for each exercise.

1. ARM-TONING EXERCISES	STARTER Sets/Reps	EXPERIENCED Sets/Reps
Triceps Extensions (page 70)	2/10	3/12
Triceps Kickbacks (page 74)	2/10	3/12
Lying Triceps Extensions (page 86)	2/10	3/12
Alternating Curls (page 71)	2/10	3/12
Hammer Curls (page 75)	2/10	3/12
Preacher Curls (page 86)	2/10	3/12

2. BUTT-FIRMING EXERCISES	STARTER Sets/Reps	EXPERIENCED Sets/Reps
Squats (page 111)	2/10	3/12
Deadlifts (page 116)	2/10	3/12
Alternating Lunges (page 115)	2/10	3/12
Stiff-Legged Deadlifts (page 111)	2/10	3/12
Alternating Back Lunges (page 119)	2/10	3/12

3. THIGH-TIGHTENING WORKOUT

The lower body may be the area that you most want to improve through target training. If your area of concern is your thighs, then try this workout. On the other hand, if you want to firm up your thighs *and* your back side, then you may consider alternating this workout with the Butt-firming Workout on Saturdays. In addition to your Lower-body Strength Training and Cardio Training, you'll be surprised by how quickly you'll make progress in firming up your target area.

Perform all sets of one exercise before moving on to the next, or perform them circuit style, where you perform one set of each exercise before returning to the first exercise for your second set. Continue working from the first exercise to the last until you have performed all sets for each exercise.

4. BODY FAT–REDUCING WORKOUT

In this workout, you perform weight exercises using a slightly lighter weight than you do on your upper- and lower-body strength-training days. Although we include a few more sets than in the strength-training workouts, you should still be able to finish the workout in 15 minutes since you won't rest between sets.

Perform the first set of the first exercise (chest presses), then move on to the next exercise (walking lunges) for the second set. Perform one set of each exercise, circuit-style, before returning to chest presses for the second round. As you perform each rep, force your body to work harder than it needs to by squeezing your target muscle. This will not only emphasize toning, but also calorie burning and ultimately body fat reduction.

3. THIGH-TIGHTENING EXERCISES	STARTER Sets/Reps	EXPERIENCED Sets/Reps
Alternating Lunges variation (page 115)	3/10	4/12
Side Lunges (page 120)	3/10	4/12
Lunges (page 119)	2/10	4/12
Alternating Back Lunges (page 119)	2/10	3/12

4. BODY FAT–REDUCING EXERCISES	STARTER Sets/Reps	EXPERIENCED Sets/Reps
Chest Presses (page 69)	2/10	3/12
Alternating Lunges variation (page 115)	2/10	3/12
Overhead Shoulder Presses (page 69)	2/10	3/12
Squats (page 111)	2/10	3/12
Dumbbell Rows (page 70)	2/10	3/12
Alternating Lunges (page 115)	2/10	3/12

SATURDAY

Target Training

5. UPPER-BODY WORKOUT

The purpose of this workout is to build muscle by allowing an extra day a week for training the primary muscle groups of the upper body. Using only one major movement (but up to five sets) for each large upper-body muscle group (chest, back and shoulders), you can stimulate more muscle building. When your goal is muscle building, use heavier weights.

6. ABS-DEVELOPING WORKOUT

To really develop amazing abs, you must invest time and effort into both your nutrition program and your training. This workout puts together many of the best abs exercises into one 15-minute workout that targets your midsection from start to finish.

5. UPPER-BODY EXERCISES	STARTER Sets/Reps	EXPERIENCED Sets/Reps
Chest Presses (page 69)	3/10	5/12
Dumbbell Rows (page 70)	3/10	5/12
Overhead Shoulder Presses (page 69)	3/10	5/12

6. ABS-DEVELOPING EXERCISES	STARTER Sets/Reps	EXPERIENCED Sets/Reps
Ball Crunches (page 71)	2/10	3/12
Cross-Body Twists (page 75)	2/10	3/12
Floor Knee-Ups (page 79)	2/10	3/12
Side Crunches (page 87)	2/10	3/12
V-Pike Raises (page 117)	2/10	3/12

7. FLEXIBILITY TARGET

While performing flexibility work once a week is far better than not performing it at all, you'll find that you get much improved results from doing flexibility work more than once a week. Choose the flexibility workout that appeals to you most and perform that for your Saturday target-training workouts (in addition to your Wednesday flexibility workouts). Also, feel free to add a few of these flexibility moves to other workouts. You can include them between sets on your Tuesday and Thursday strength workouts, or before or after your cardio workouts on Mondays and Fridays.

8. CARDIO WORKOUT

If your biggest training concern is your cardio-vascular health (and the benefits associated with this type of training), you may opt to include a third day of cardio training each week. Choose the type of cardio training that appeals to you most and perform that for your Saturday workouts (in addition to Mondays and Fridays). You can opt to do the same cardio exercise three times a week, or you can choose a different type. If cardio fitness is your ultimate goal, then you may find that cross-training (performing more than one type of cardio exercise each week) is the best way to accomplish this.

Sunday

mind/body workouts

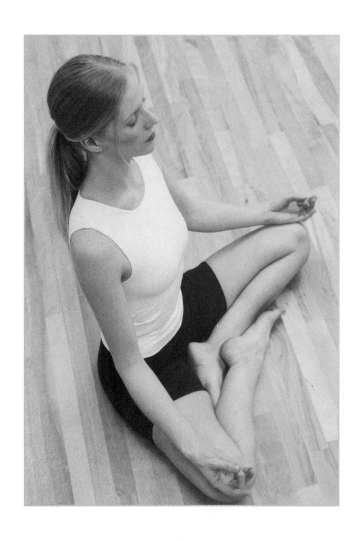

To make the most of your Mind/Body Training, choose an option that allows you to relax—not all of these workouts will be appropriate for everyone. For instance, if you don't like being touched by strangers, you won't be able to derive the full benefits from a massage. If you get bored and impatient when you take a bath, then you should also seek out another option—being bored is not the same as being relaxed.

A sign that you're relaxing is when your breathing slows, becoming deep and even. Your heart rate should also drop a bit. When you're relaxed, you should be able to clear your mind of all your daily concerns, yet still maintain consciousness. During this time, focus your mind on the relaxation of your body.

OPTION 1	Get a Massage
OPTION 2	Soak in a Bathtub
OPTION 3	Relax in a Hot Tub
OPTION 4	Sweat in a Steam Room
OPTION 5	Perform a Slow Stretch
OPTION 6	Meditate or Pray

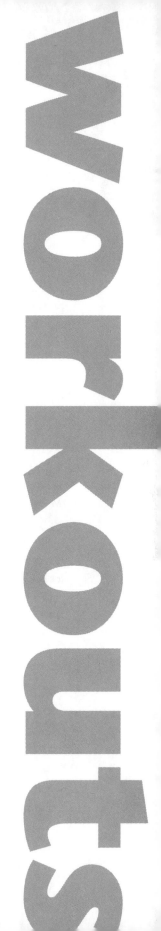

workouts

Mind/Body

1. GET A MASSAGE

A massage promotes relaxation in several ways. The masseuse applies direct pressure to your muscles so that they gradually relax. By slowing your breathing and learning to breathe with the pressure given by the masseuse, you also enhance total body relaxation. Many masseuses will tell you when to inhale and exhale at times throughout the massage.

Be sure to tell the masseuse which areas are tightest, or the areas that you would find most relaxing to have massaged.

2. SOAK IN A BATHTUB

Warm water can be very relaxing, but it can also sap your energy—often this is a better option at night rather than first thing in the morning. Check with your doctor that this is a safe option for you, especially before taking a bath in hot or cold water for an extended period of time.

During your bath, focus on slowing your heart rate and breathing deeply and slowly. This will help deepen your relaxation and provide more of the restorative effects of a Mind/Body Workout.

3. RELAX IN A HOT TUB

Warm water can be very relaxing, but it can also sap your energy—soaking in hot water is a better option at night rather than first thing in the morning. If you plan to do this first thing in the morning, you might seek out a cooler temperature of water.

Check with your doctor to make certain this is a safe option for you, especially before using a hot tub with an extreme temperature for an extended period of time. During your time in the hot tub, focus on slowing your heart rate and breathing deeply and slowly. This will help deepen your relaxation and provide more of the restorative effects of a Mind/Body Workout.

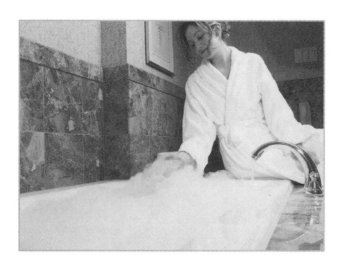

4. SWEAT IN A STEAM ROOM

Using a steam room can be very relaxing, but it can also sap your energy so plan your day accordingly. Often, the temperature of a steam room is quite hot. Check with your doctor to make certain this is a safe option for you. You should also start slowly, spending only a few minutes in a steam room, allowing your body to grow accustomed to this new physical stimulation.

During your time in the steam room, focus on slowing your heart rate and breathing deeply and slowly. This will help deepen your relaxation and provide more of the restorative effects of a Mind/Body Workout.

5. PERFORM A SLOW STRETCH

If you are taking a class (yoga or Pilates) or performing a slow stretch on your own, you should emphasize the relaxing qualities of the movement. Often, yoga or Pilates classes can be full workouts in and of themselves. Find a class that emphasizes relaxation, but if none is available, take one of the easier classes and move slowly, staying focused on relaxation over deep stretching.

During any form of stretching for relaxation, you should emphasize slow, deep breathing, and slow movements, holding your stretches for several seconds to as long as a minute or two.

6. MEDITATE OR PRAY

While your prayers and meditations should be of your own making, do try to keep focused on how the spiritual element connects to your physical well-being. This will help you get the most from your Mind/Body Training. Emphasize deep, even breaths while you meditate or pray as a way to enhance the mind/body element.

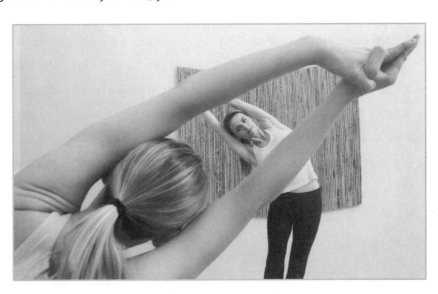

Continue Your Progress

BUILDING LONGER WORKOUTS

As you gain more experience on your Fit in 15 program, you may find that on some days you want to work out longer than 15 minutes. Try these tips:

ADD MORE REPS AND SETS. If you want to increase upper-body work, add another set or two of each exercise, and/or add a few more reps to each set (e.g., instead of doing 12 reps of biceps curls, try 15). Note that you may need more recovery time between sets.

ADD MORE WEIGHT. Rather than adding more reps, perform the same number of reps with additional weight. This may also require more rest between sets.

ADD MORE EXERCISES. You can add another exercise or two from one of the other workout options to the workout you like best.

PERFORM LONGER CARDIO SESSIONS. For cardiovascular training, simply perform your exercise of choice for a longer period of time, but remember to build up slowly.

COMBINE DIFFERENT TYPES OF EXERCISE. Cross-training stimulates your muscles a little differently, giving you a more well-rounded workout. In the middle of your workout, consider switching from a treadmill to a stationary bike. Try ten minutes on each.

COMBINE DIFFERENT TYPES OF TRAINING. If you're content to perform 15 minutes of strength training but have some time for another type of training, then take a five- or ten-minute brisk walk. Cross-training will help you burn more calories as well as encourage better overall fitness. Keep in mind that you'll get benefits regardless of whether you exercise all at once or at different intervals throughout the day. For instance, you can perform strength training in the morning before work; on your lunch break, you can also add in an invigorating walk.

CHANGE YOUR PROGRAM

For the best results from your Fit in 15 program, consider changing your program about every eight weeks. For instance, if your goal is to tone your arms, it may seem logical to focus on them at all times, including an extra arms workout on every Target Training Saturday. But you'll get better results for them and your whole body by changing your program. So do the arm-toning program for eight weeks, then switch to another Target Training workout for the next six to eight weeks. Return to the arm-toning program for the next eight weeks, then try the flexibility program for six weeks before going back to the arm-toning program. This type of cycling allows for target improvements while also enhancing total fitness.

GET FIT WITH INTENSITY

One of the most important components in improving your fitness level is the intensity with which you perform your Fit in 15 program. Many people think that using more weight or more sets or running faster or stretching deeper is the key, but all of these really rely on increased intensity—a basic element in continuing to make improvements.

Working with intensity means putting as much effort as you can into your exercise. For instance, when you perform a crunch in your core training, try to force your abs to "crunch" down even harder than is needed to raise your upper body. This additional effort sends the message to your brain and body that you are asking more of it, and your body will respond by adapting. In this case, the added intensity will help to develop even more definition in your abdominal muscles.

The same is true for weight exercises. While you can go through the motions of lifting a weight, you'll get better results by putting even more effort into each rep of each exercise. Contract your target muscle even harder than is necessary to perform the rep. This recruits more muscle fibers, thus developing more muscle tone and definition.

VARY YOUR INTENSITY

While using increased intensity is one of the keys to getting fit, you also want to work out at different intensity levels during different workouts. Many people always work out at the same level of intensity for every workout—either easy, moderate or hard. But there are huge advantages to varying the intensity of the work you do from one session to the next. It's okay to really break a sweat on your upper-body and core strength-training day, then go for an Easy-Does-It Walk on your cardio day. Similarly, you may want to really get your heart rate up on your cardio day, then make your strength day and your flexibility days a little easier the next week.

Variation in intensity allows for better progress by not letting your body adapt as easily to one type of stimulation. Even marathoners will include short, easy jogs in their training on some days. This helps their bodies better accommodate to the immense demands of marathon running than a daily long-distance run does.

These two concepts—increasing intensity and varying intensity— are compatible with one another. By working out at different intensity levels from one workout to the next, you are also better able to increase intensity from your easy training days to your more intense training days.

About the Author

STEVEN STIEFEL, the author of *Weights on the Ball Workout*, has been a health and fitness writer for over a decade and is currently the nutrition editor at *FLEX Magazine*. Previously, he was a contributing editor at *Men's Fitness* magazine. He also writes articles for *Muscle & Fitness*, *HERS* and other health and fitness publications. Steven earned his master's degrees at the University of Arizona and the University of Southern California. His short fiction has appeared in *The Georgia Review*, *McSweeney's* and other publications. In addition to his writing career, Steven also serves as Chief Creative Officer for Ronick Productions, a feature film company located in Los Angeles.